Gut Goals

About the Author

Beth Rosen, MS, RD, CDN is a weight-inclusive registered dietitian specializing in gastrointestinal (GI) nutrition and disordered eating, who has been working in the field of nutrition for 30 years. In her private practice, Beth helps clients find relief from digestive disorders such as irritable bowel disease (IBS), small intestinal bacterial overgrowth (SIBO), gastroparesis, gastroesophageal reflux disease, and celiac disease. Beth herself suffered from gut issues for years before she fought for a diagnosis of post-infectious IBS by advocating for herself and educating herself on GI issues. She lives on Long Island with her husband, who has microscopic colitis, her daughter, who has lactose intolerance, and their two dogs with food intolerances. Miraculously, her son manages to tolerate all foods to this day.

Overcoming Common Problems

Gut Goals

A Practical Plan for Managing IBS

BETH ROSEN, MS, RD, CDN

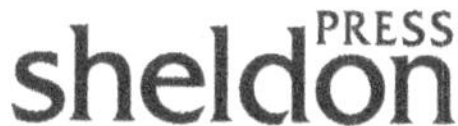

First published in Great Britain by Sheldon Press in 2026
An imprint of John Murray Press

SRD

A CIP catalogue record for this title is available from the British Library and the Library of Congress Control Number.

Trade Paperback ISBN 978 1 399 82137 7
ebook ISBN 978 1 399 82139 1

Typeset by KnowledgeWorks Global Ltd.

Printed and bound in India by Manipal Technologies Limited, Manipal

John Murray Press policy is to use papers that are natural, renewable and recyclable products and made from wood grown in sustainable forests. The logging and manufacturing processes are expected to conform to the environmental regulations of the country of origin.

John Murray Press
Carmelite House
50 Victoria Embankment
London EC4Y 0DZ

Sheldon Press
Hachette Book Group
123 South Broad Street
Ste 2750
Philadelphia, PA 19109, USA

www.sheldonpress.co.uk

John Murray Press, part of Hodder & Stoughton Limited
An Hachette UK company

For Eli and Amelia

Contents

1
Introduction
My IBS Story and Philosophy on Care

If you are reading this page then most likely you a) have irritable bowel syndrome (IBS), b) know someone who does, or c) are having some gastrointestinal (GI) issues that are troubling you and you are looking for help. Well then, this book is for you. IBS is no joke, and it's not something you can self-diagnose, nor is it a diagnosis of "we don't know what this is so let's just call it irritable bowel syndrome." It's important that before you treat any GI symptom on your own, you seek care from a physician (ideally a gastroenterologist) and get a proper diagnosis, or at the very least rule out diseases that need specific specialized care (more on this in Chapter 4).

As a registered dietitian (RD) for over 30 years, I have worked with many clients to improve their symptoms and quality of life through both dietary and non-diet interventions. My ultimate goal is that these pages provide you with a framework to seek care, advocate for yourself, and find the same digestive peace that I and so many of my clients have found.

Yes, you read that right, I said *"I."*

Not only am I a registered dietitian, I'm a patient, too.

Everybody Poops

Before I tell you my IBS story though, I want to talk about one of my favorite subjects—poop. In fact, I am going to be talking a lot about bowel movements, stool, number twos, dropping the kids off at the pool, or whatever you call it, throughout the pages in this book. You might say I talk a shit-ton about shit—its size, shape, color, and consistency. Your poop can tell you a lot about your gut health and it can offer your healthcare providers a clue as to what might be causing your symptoms (more on this in Chapter 3).

Many people are embarrassed when asked to talk about their poop and avoid alerting their healthcare providers about what they see in the bowl or on the paper when they wipe because they think it is uncouth. Omitting your poop story from the information you share with your doctors may lead to a delay in diagnosis and care, or misdiagnosis and ineffective care. If you are among these people, I have a secret to share with you: Everybody poops! There are even children's books about it.

Getting comfortable with bodily functions and deciphering dysfunctions is an integral part of understanding your body and how it works so that you can get care when you need it. In fact, you know your body best, so we rely on you to share your crap chronicles with us, along with all of your GI symptom details. Doctors, dietitians, and other healthcare providers have tools like blood tests, scans, and nutrition plans, but we won't know if we are helping you heal, recover, or manage your symptoms and diagnoses without your complete input and feedback. After all, you live in your body, so you know it best, and you are the keeper of your IBS story.

My IBS Story

In 2010, after a recent move to Connecticut, my then six-year-old daughter was hospitalized with pneumonia after having swine flu. She and I spent two nights in the hospital—she in the bed, me in a chair. At the time, I was on a course of antibiotics for a minor infection and thought nothing of the potential impact they might have on my microbiome. In fact, I don't think I *ever* considered my microbiome prior to my IBS diagnosis (more on the microbiome in Chapter 2).

A few weeks later, I came down with a "stomach bug" that began with abdominal cramping, pain, and urgent diarrhea. I assumed it was something I ate (as many people do) and began cutting things out of my diet to rid my body of the culprit. My symptoms continued: excruciating gut pain, urgent diarrhea that woke me up in the early morning and persisted all day, and spasming throughout my lower abdomen. So I removed more and more foods and food groups from my diet.

At the recommendation of a family member, I took a food sensitivity test (more on these in Chapter 4) and eliminated 40 foods based on the results. My diet was now made up of the flesh of baked potatoes, pita chips, and plain grilled chicken. My energy was low, I was unintentionally losing weight, and my symptoms persisted uncontrollably. I was urgently moving my bowels more frequently each day until one day the pain was so severe, and the diarrhea seemed so endless, that I needed to go to the emergency room. While there, they just rehydrated me, gave me something for the pain, and referred me to a gastroenterologist, who was able to see me the next day.

After a stool test, I was diagnosed with *Clostridioides difficile*, an infection known as *C.diff*, which causes diarrhea and inflammation of the colon. I was put on antibiotics and told that I would be back to normal within two weeks.

After two weeks, my symptoms weren't as intense, but they persisted. The gastroenterologist suggested that I eliminate gluten, dairy, and eggs to alleviate my symptoms. This proved to be difficult and impacted my ability to eat socially and prepare meals and snacks for my family without becoming a short-order cook. While these changes did not help, I did not return these foods to my eating pattern for fear that they might still be part of the problem.

Then I received a phone call from the Centers for Disease Control and Prevention (CDC). Apparently, they keep track of *C. diff* diagnoses and asked me a series of questions to ascertain where I might have contracted it. Lo and behold, the CDC said without hesitation that my two-night stay in the hospital while on antibiotics was the impetus. *C. diff* is extremely contagious and can easily be passed from patient to patient (or mom) in hospitals via healthcare staff, shared bathrooms, and even the privacy curtains that hang in patient rooms. The best way to avoid contracting it is proper handwashing and cleaning surfaces with antimicrobial products.

I returned to the gastroenterologist and he suggested I have an endoscopy to look for what else might be causing my pain and discomfort. When I awoke, he told me that he did not see anything (nor did he biopsy anything which would have definitively ruled out celiac disease), and he offered me toast with butter (uh, what about no gluten or dairy?). Confused and sad, I had no more answers or solutions than I did before the endoscopy, nor ways to manage my symptoms. When I pressed him for more help, he told me that I had post-infectious IBS (PI-IBS) and my symptoms would clear within two years. I was devastated that I would have to live with pain and urgent diarrhea for that long.

After 18 months, I switched doctors to see if perhaps another practitioner might have solutions. The new gastroenterologist sent me for stool testing, a blood test to rule out celiac disease, and a colonoscopy. While the colonoscopy revealed nothing other than inflammation, the blood test indicated that I had non-celiac gluten sensitivity (NCGS) and the stool test indicated that I *still* had *C. diff*. No wonder my symptoms were not improving! I was treated again with antibiotics, and again my symptoms improved slightly, but I certainly did not feel better. I had a hard time believing that I had NCGS. After initially eliminating gluten, I had added it back after my endoscopy the year before, so I went home and made pasta for dinner. Big mistake! My belly swelled and ached for the rest of the night and into the morning. Since that day, I have avoided eating gluten-containing foods.

I visited the gastroenterologist every six weeks for the recommended follow-ups, but there was nothing they could do for me. My parents begged me to switch providers, this time to one in New York City. That doctor sent me for lactose intolerance testing and small intestinal bowel syndrome (SIBO) breath testing, and I tested positive for both (more on this in Chapter 4). I went on another round of antibiotics and avoided dairy as recommended. While we were discussing my treatment plan, the gastroenterologist took not one but two phone calls. I sat in her office, listening to her talk about other patients with a colleague. Instead of apologizing for the disruption of our time, she said their cases were more serious and urgent than mine.

Time to find yet another doctor.

While on the hunt, I began to have bladder pain in addition to the PI-IBS and SIBO-related discomfort. I was referred to a urologist who diagnosed me with interstitial cystitis (IC). IC is a chronic, painful condition where the bladder is overly sensitive to being filled with urine.

I continued my search for a doctor who might listen to my issues and teach me how to manage them. A friend recommended one that she worked with (she was a nurse and worked in the research department at Yale). I didn't want a repeat of all of the testing and recommendations that I had received from my previous doctors, so I wrote a detailed history of what I had been through over the past two years.

I went for my first visit and met the kindest, most attentive physician I have ever encountered. He sat and reviewed my history with me, asking me questions and validating my frustration and perpetual discomfort with and within my body. Then he told me something that I wasn't ready to hear: *I had irritable bowel syndrome and it was never going to go away.* I knew that there were worse diagnoses I could have received in my lifetime, but I couldn't believe it. *C. diff* had triggered a chronic illness in my gastrointestinal system that I was now going to have to learn how to live with for the rest of my life. I cried right there in the office. The doctor assured me that although there was no cure, he had plenty of ways to bring my pain and discomfort levels from a seven or eight out of ten to a two or a three. I trusted him. He validated my experiences and gave me tools to manage each symptom I shared with him.

If you were keeping count, I saw four gastroenterologists over the course of two years before having an appropriate diagnosis and someone to guide me through evidence-based management tools for my symptoms. I started to find relief from my IBS, but it took a lot of time and trial and error to reach my "new normal" of living with a chronic illness. I spent two years blaming food for my symptoms when restriction might have been exacerbating them. I lived with pain, bloating, lack of trust in my body, and urgent loose stools for years until my doctor partnered with me to find what eased my symptoms. IBS has not been an easy ride. I still have flares where my symptoms return, but now I have tools to help me manage my symptoms and reduce their frequency, severity, and duration.

Why You Won't Find Weight Loss Prescribed in This Book or in My Practice

Weight loss is often touted as a panacea for various health conditions, including GI diseases like gastroesophageal reflux disease (GERD) and metabolic dysfunction-associated steatotic liver disease (MASLD, aka fatty liver disease). Many medical professionals are quick to prescribe it as a remedy by telling clients to "just lose weight and exercise." However, when we look at the research, we see a different, and potentially dangerous, picture. Some studies may correlate weight with health outcomes, but they often fail to see that the underlying health behaviors are what truly drive improvements in health.

Think of it this way: You are told to lose weight and exercise to improve your cholesterol numbers. So, you begin a walking regimen, add in a salad with your dinner, grab some fruit for a snack after lunch, and change your white bread to whole wheat. At your next doctor visit, you've indeed lost a few pounds and your cholesterol has dropped a few points. You are praised for the weight loss because it "worked" and are encouraged to keep up the good work.

But who is to say that the decrease in cholesterol was due to the weight loss and not to the added fiber from fruits, veggies, and whole grains? Unless studies specifically control for calorie restriction on its own for weight loss versus adding health behaviors, like increasing fiber-rich foods and movement, the lower cholesterol is only *correlated* with weight loss and it cannot definitively be proven that it was *caused* by weight loss. Correlation is a connection between two things while causation is a cause and effect between two things.

Here's an example of the difference between correlation and causation. A man with yellow teeth develops lung cancer, and there seems to be a growing trend of people having yellow teeth and being diagnosed with lung cancer. So, people start doing everything they can to reduce their risk of lung cancer by getting their teeth whitened and avoiding foods like berries and coffee that can stain the teeth. The yellow teeth and lung cancer connection is a correlation. When research is done on this relationship to see what other factors may be present that might correlate with or cause lung cancer, they find that those with yellow teeth also smoke cigarettes, and for those who smoke, their risk for cancer is increased. For those with yellow teeth who smoke and make efforts to whiten their teeth, a decrease in cancer risk is not seen. The researchers also find that there are study participants with yellow teeth that don't smoke and don't develop lung cancer at the rates at which the smokers with yellow teeth and white teeth do. They conclude that smoking causes cancer and that yellow teeth is one correlation with lung cancer, but because smokers who whiten their teeth are still at an increased risk of cancer, yellow teeth is only a correlation with cancer and with smoking.

Behaviors such as regular exercise, incorporating fiber-rich foods into your diet, smoking cessation, and managing stress levels can all lead to positive health outcomes. These behaviors, referred to as "health-promoting behaviors," can be the catalyst for changes in health *independent of* weight loss, meaning that you can partake in these behaviors to improve your health without losing weight and you will still benefit from those behaviors ... to a degree.

What is often overlooked is the impact that genetics and the social determinants of health (for example, access to healthcare, socioeconomic status, race) play in the determination of who develops reflux, fatty liver disease, diabetes, etc. These factors influence our health far beyond what diet and exercise alone can do. In fact, the amount of control we have over our health is about 29 percent—that means that approximately 71 percent of our health is in the hands of our genes, how much money we have, and if we live near places that have lots of skilled healthcare providers. I tell you this not to dissuade you from participating in health-promoting behaviors but to inform you so that you are aware that your IBS and many other chronic illnesses are not within your total control. Changing your weight or living in a thin body is not a guarantee that you will be disease-free. There is not one disease—not cancer, diabetes, or reflux—that is only diagnosed in people living in larger bodies.

Let's say that you believe (as many do) that living in a smaller body is the key to health. How would you go about being and staying smaller? Research tells us that the pursuit of weight loss through restrictive diets or intense exercise regimens is frequently unsustainable in the long term; the vast majority—anywhere from 88 percent to 95 percent—of individuals who embark on a diet will ultimately regain the weight they lost within three to five years. Of those people who regain the weight, two thirds will gain more than they initially lost (Tylka et al., 2014). This phenomenon, known as weight cycling or yo-yo dieting, not only fails to deliver lasting weight loss but also comes with a host of negative consequences.

Weight cycling has been linked to increased inflammation, which subsequently increases the risk of developing various chronic diseases. It's important to note that the emotional toll of repeatedly losing and regaining weight can be profound, contributing to heightened levels of stress and leaving people vulnerable to disordered eating patterns and eating disorder diagnoses. Assigning blame to one's body size for health concerns perpetuates harmful stereotypes and biases. It is important that healthcare providers prioritize addressing symptoms and improving overall well-being rather than fixating on weight. It is downright wrong to diagnose one's fatness as the cause of their disease in one person while offering a thin person medical interventions to manage or treat the same disease. Your healthcare professionals should emphasize the adoption of sustainable, health-promoting behaviors that can yield significant improvements in health outcomes without the detrimental effects associated with weight-focused interventions. Look for these providers—they exist.

A Note on Language

You may have noticed that while I was talking about bodies, I didn't use the words "overweight" or "obese," and that was intentional. These words are based on the Body Mass Index (BMI), which many experts consider to be flawed. The BMI doesn't accurately measure health risks for populations or individuals and is based on height versus weight without any consideration for conditioned muscles, age, gender, or race.

Sticks and Stones May Break Bones, But Words Can Lead to Weight Bias

Language plays a crucial role here—simply by their definitions, these terms can reinforce biases against people with bigger bodies. For instance, "obesity" comes from a Latin phrase meaning "eaten itself fat," implying that everyone with a larger body is that way due to lacking willpower, overeating, laziness, or neglecting their health. Similarly, "overweight" suggests that there's an ideal weight for every height and exceeding it carries the same stereotypes as "obesity." I and many of my colleagues in the fat liberation movement have embraced the term "fat" as a neutral descriptor, akin to "tall" or "muscular." Other preferred terms include "in a larger/bigger body" or "at a higher weight." To reduce the risk of contributing to or reinforcing weight stigma or bias, I will not use the "o" words when referring to bodies and I hope you will consider doing the same in your everyday life.

My Care Philosophy

My experience was the catalyst for the pivot in my career as a registered dietitian and in my resolve: to support and guide my clients with GI issues by helping them seek out skilled practitioners, share their symptoms, and advocate for equitable and appropriate care so that they can improve their quality of life and once again have digestive peace. You might say that these are my gut goals.

Now, you've gotten to know a little about me and my weight-inclusive approach to treating my clients, but I don't know you (though I would very much like to!). You may have IBS or think you do, but you may also have heart disease, thyroid issues, autoimmune diseases, or an eating disorder. Because I cannot begin to know you through the pages of this book, I cannot be your personal registered dietitian merely by what I provide in these pages. What I will share with you will help you manage your symptoms, reduce the duration, intensity, and frequency of your flares, and offer you hope that while living with IBS you can still enjoy all that life has to offer. None of my advice will focus on losing weight because this isn't the best way to improve health. Instead, by thinking about the larger picture of health and focusing on health-promoting habits, we can safely work toward feeling better and being flare-free.

However, this does not replace working with your gastroenterologist or any other healthcare practitioners in real life. I state this so that you are aware that my goal is to avoid harming you or exacerbating your co-occurring illnesses. When you decide to apply my recommendations, please first look at the big picture of your health and collaborate with your healthcare team to ensure that solving your digestive issues won't trigger a hiccup with your other health issues.

Let's get started!

2
How the Gut Works (for People without IBS)

Before we can begin to understand what is going on in a digestive system that has IBS, we must review how the gut works for people without digestive issues. The terms *digestive system* and *gut* are interchangeable and reference the parts of your body that are involved in turning your food into energy, nourishment for your microbiome, and waste that leaves your body. Let's take a trip through the digestive system to see exactly what happens when you eat.

The Land of Chew and Swallow: Mouth and Esophagus

You might not be aware of what's happening when you take a bite of your favorite food, but it goes through a wild ride in order to extract nutrients and give you energy. That mouthful of deliciousness starts its journey by going through three steps of swallowing (called deglutition) to get from your mouth to your stomach.

The first phase is called the oral phase. This phase begins with chewing, where your teeth and tongue break food into smaller pieces. Different teeth have different jobs: incisors cut, canines tear, and molars grind. The masseter—aka the jaw muscle—is the strongest muscle for its size in the body and helps crush food.

Salivary glands produce saliva while chewing is happening. Saliva contains water, mucin (a protein that helps with lubrication), and enzymes that start breaking down carbohydrates in your mouth. As you chew, food mixes with saliva and breaks down into a moist, soft ball of food called a bolus. The tongue helps to push the bolus to the back of the throat to ready it for the next phase of swallowing.

The second phase, called the pharyngeal phase, starts with the food bolus hitting your throat and triggering a cascade of events

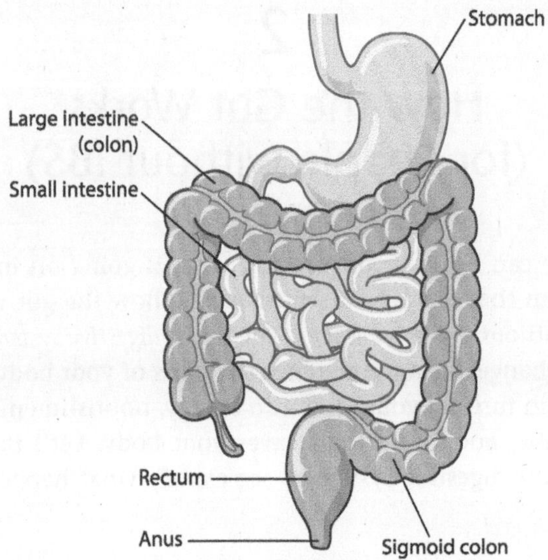

Figure 2.1 Features of the digestive system

that stops it from going up your nose or down your windpipe. Instead, the food bolus is guided to the top of your esophagus.

This begins the third phase of swallowing called the esophageal phase. Wave-like contractions push the bolus down toward the stomach via the esophagus. There is a muscle at the bottom of the esophagus called the lower esophageal sphincter. It opens up when food is on its way down and quickly closes once the food enters to prevent stomach acid from bubbling up into the esophagus.

Digestion Time: The Stomach

The purpose of digestion is to break down the food bolus further so that nutrients can be absorbed in the small intestine. Before the food reaches the small intestine, it goes through digestion in the stomach in three stages. It begins with mechanical and chemical digestion: the stomach churns food with stomach acid and enzymes to methodically break it down. The stomach is very acidic and contains several types of cells responsible for the next stage of digestion, which involves breaking down proteins, killing bacteria, and producing mucus to protect the stomach lining from acid. The final stage controls the release of the stomach contents into the small intestine. Fluids are released faster than solids, now called chyme.

The Long and Winding Road: The Small Intestine

The small intestine is the longest part of our digestive tract at an average of 22 feet, or 7 meters, in length. Like the esophagus, the small intestine moves food with continuous contractions and mixing movements to ensure it makes contact with digestive enzymes and bile. The small intestine is lined with *villi*, tiny finger-like structures that increase the surface area and facilitate absorption of vitamins, minerals, and other nutrients.

There are three sections of the small intestine:

- duodenum
- jejunum
- ileum.

The first section of the small intestine is the duodenum where iron, calcium, magnesium, and folate are absorbed. The second section, the jejunum, absorbs the bulk of our nutrients including simple sugars, fatty acids, amino acids, and vitamins A, D, E, K, and C, and B-complex vitamins. The ileum is the shortest of the small intestine sections and is responsible for the uptake of vitamin B12.

Accessories are Everything: Pancreas, Liver, and Gallbladder

Let's back up briefly to explain the origins of the enzymes needed for complete digestion. The cells of the stomach produce all the enzymes it needs to break down the food bolus enough to move it onto the small intestine. But the small intestine can't complete digestion and absorption all on its own—it needs help from the accessory organs, namely the pancreas, liver, and gallbladder.

The pancreas releases digestive enzymes and bicarbonate to further break down the chyme and neutralize the stomach acid.

It also manages blood sugar through its controlled release of insulin and glucagon.

The liver and gallbladder work hand in hand. The liver makes bile, which helps digest fats, and the gallbladder stores bile and releases it into the small intestine when needed. If you no longer have a gallbladder, no worries! Our livers are so smart that they will get to know how much fat you typically take in during a meal and release enough fat-digesting enzymes when you eat.

Almost There: The Large Intestine, aka the Colon

Once digestion and absorption of nutrients are completed, what's left makes its way through a gate called the ileocecal valve. This valve keeps small intestine contents in the small intestine until all the nutrients have been extracted, and it prevents the microbes living in the large intestine from migrating up into the small intestine where they don't belong.

The colon is not as long as the small intestine, but it is wider in diameter, thus earning the name "large intestine." It's about 5 feet long, or 150 centimeters, and has a few sections:

- the ascending colon, which runs up the right side of your abdomen
- the transverse colon, which runs across your abdomen
- the descending colon, which runs down the left side of your abdomen
- the sigmoid colon, which is at the very bottom of your large intestine and curves to meet up with your rectum.

The colon mainly absorbs water and electrolytes, leaving behind solid waste (aka feces, poop, number twos). There are up to 100 trillion microbes living in our large intestine that produce B-complex vitamins, vitamin K, and short-chain fatty acids (SCFAs) that offer myriad health benefits (more on this in the microbiome section).

Last Stop: The Rectum and the Anus

When water and electrolytes are removed and form the feces, we don't immediately run to the bathroom. Instead, the rectum stores feces until there is enough to cause distension and signal expulsion. That distension or pressure is what you feel when you need to move your bowels, but have no fear, they will not move themselves in a healthy digestive system.

There are internal and external anal sphincters, which is the same type of muscular doorway that you find between the esophagus and the stomach and between the stomach and the small intestine. These sphincters control the release of feces, working with muscles located in your pelvic floor to ensure you choose when you go and when you hold it. When you are seated on the porcelain throne (aka the toilet), those muscles will relax and contract to move stool out of your body and into the bowl.

Time Travel

Everyone chews, swallows, digests, and defecates at different rates, especially those with IBS. But for those without IBS, the entire digestive process can take between 24 and 72 hours and depends on a few factors.

Diet is the most obvious factor in digestive time travel. Foods that are high in fiber temporarily slow digestion in the stomach but speed up digestion in the intestines.

Fiber is found in:

- fruits and vegetables
- nuts and seeds
- whole grains
- beans
- legumes.

The amount of fluid we drink also dictates the ease of digestion. When we are adequately hydrated—whether it be from water, juice, carbonated beverages, or tea—things move *smoothly*, if you know what I mean.

Movement, exercise, or having an active lifestyle all play a role in promoting healthy digestion. Physical activity stimulates muscle contractions in your digestive tract that keep things moving and improve blood flow, which makes the absorption of vitamins, minerals, and other nutrients more efficient.

Microbes, Microbiota, Microbiome, Oh My!

Imagine a bustling city inside of you where different types of organisms live and work in harmony with each other toward their goal of providing you with optimal health, while also protecting you from pathogenic (disease-causing) organisms. This magical metropolis is called your *gut microbiome*. The gut microbiome is inhabited by *gut microbiota*, which include microscopic *microbes* such as bacteria, viruses, fungi, protozoa, and archaea. These critters work both alone and in groups to create byproducts, called *metabolites*, that influence digestion, immune function, and even brain activity. Together, the microbes in the microbiota plus the metabolites they make are considered your gut microbiome. You have other microbiomes in other parts of your body like your skin and vagina, but for the sake of this book, I will use the term *microbiome* to mean the gut microbiome.

Your microbiome is responsible for a number of functions that impact both your gut health and the health of other parts of your body.

Digestion and Nutrient Absorption

Remember that part where you learned about the large intestine and all the goings-on during digestion and absorption? Well, the microbiome assists in the breakdown of complex carbohydrates, proteins, and fats that our digestive system cannot process on its own. It can also create vitamins through a process called synthesis. Certain gut bacteria are responsible for making essential vitamins, including vitamin K and B vitamins (B12, biotin, folate), which are vital for blood clotting, energy production, and cell metabolism. The other vitamins and minerals we need for optimal health come from the food we eat and are absorbed into the bloodstream during digestion.

When complex carbohydrates go through the process of deconstruction, microbes feed on fiber, ferment it (which is how gas is formed), and break it down into short-chain fatty acids. SCFAs are crucial for gut health as they provide energy to colon cells and regulate inflammation. They also support intestinal barrier function at the cellular level, and can be used as an energy source by our bodies. Microbial metabolites play a role in the breakdown of fat and influence fat storage both in how much and where on the body.

Gut Barrier Maintenance

You might have heard of "leaky gut" before. While not an official diagnosis, it describes when the barrier cells of the intestinal wall become inflamed and are no longer tightly packed together. A tight cell structure regulates what passes into the bloodstream; it keeps the contents of the colon inside the colon. When this structure loosens due to inflammation and becomes "leaky," undigested food particles can pass through and trigger an immune response.

These leaking spaces continue if our immune system recognizes the inflamed barrier cells and food particles as foreign bodies and sets off an immune response. The immune response can persist in a vicious cycle with barrier permeability and may lead to the immune system attacking the body's tissues. This process can put us at risk for chronic inflammation and autoimmune disease development.

Protecting Against Pathogens

Imagine trying to climb a rock wall and all of a sudden an avalanche of slime comes barreling toward you, knocking you back down to the ground. That slime now coats the rock wall, making it slippery and hard to grip onto the edges and progress back up the wall. This is what some of the beneficial bacteria do in our intestines: they produce mucus to coat the intestinal wall, making it almost impossible for pathogens (disease-causing organisms like bacteria or viruses) to gain access to our tight junctions and cause trouble. Incidentally, this mucus also helps lubricate the intestinal tract, making it easier to move waste toward the exit.

Beneficial microbes protect against pathogens through something called *competitive exclusion*. Competitive exclusion is like survival of the fittest: microbes outcompete pathogens for nutrients and attachment sites on the gut lining, which protects the lining and prevents infections. Some microbes produce antimicrobial compounds that impact the growth of certain pathogenic microbes. It's like they know what kryptonite to make and who it will work against. Amazing!

Immune System Regulation

The gut microbiome plays a key role in the development of our immune system when we are young. It teaches the immune system to distinguish between harmful pathogens and harmless or beneficial microbes and their metabolites. It also modulates the activity of immune cells. This means that it ensures that the response to a pathogen is the necessary attack scenario needed to rid the body of that pathogen. If the response is too small, it can lead to an infection; if it is too big, over time it can lead to an autoimmune disease. This delicate balance is what keeps us well even when we are not aware of a pathogen like a cold bug.

Gut–Brain Axis

You might have been told that your GI symptoms are all in your head. First, we know that's not true. What you feel is valid and should be met with a concerted effort to find a solution by your healthcare provider. Second, it's a little true. The gut and brain communicate bidirectionally through the gut–brain axis, which encompasses the gut, brain, and vagus nerve, which runs from the brain to the large intestine. The gut and the brain send signals along this axis about hunger and fullness, when you need to move your bowels, and when you are experiencing anxiety or feeling bloated.

This game of telephone involves two parts. To begin, the microbes produce neurotransmitters like serotonin and dopamine, which play a role in mood regulation, stress response, and cognitive functions. Then, the vagus nerve is influenced by the microbial metabolites. If the microbes are producing too many or too few neurotransmitters, or the metabolites are causing a glitch in vagus nerve signaling, we can have a miscommunication between the brain and the gut. IBS falls into the category of disorders of the gut–brain interaction (DGBI) because our GI symptoms are directly impacted by the signaling to and from our brain.

Keeping the Little Guys Happy

While our microbiome plays a significant role in our gut health by supporting digestion, influencing metabolism, and synthesizing essential vitamins, its health depends on us. Microbes produce metabolites and those metabolites help to create a diverse and balanced microbial community. They rely on us to provide nutrients for them and avoid disrupting metabolite production from the foods we consume to the medications we take. A diet rich in varied forms of fiber from fruits, vegetables, nuts, seeds, and whole grains promotes the production of beneficial metabolites like SCFAs that provide energy to the colon and support its immune function. Conversely, taking antibiotics when we don't need them can kill off the good guys and reduce the production of metabolites, throwing the microbiome into imbalance or dysbiosis. Of course, taking all medications as prescribed might also help to reduce the likelihood of dysbiosis.

Understanding how the gut and the microbiome function in a healthy digestive system is essential before delving into how IBS can disrupt them. The digestive system works in a harmonious sequence to convert food into energy, nourish the microbiome, and eliminate waste. Each section of the digestive tract plays a specialized role in this intricate process. The gut microbiome plays a pivotal role in maintaining gut health by assisting with digesting food, synthesizing essential vitamins, and producing short-chain fatty acids and other metabolites that ensure a balanced and efficient working system. Understanding and nurturing this inner ecosystem can lead to improved health and prevention of various diseases. Now that you are familiar with it, let's look at what happens when things go awry.

3

What is IBS?

Now that we know how our digestive tract is supposed to work, we can talk about what's going on inside your gut ... and your brain. Irritable bowel syndrome is not just a disorder of your GI tract, it is also a disorder of communication between your gut and your brain. It falls under the classification of a disorder of the gut–brain interaction. IBS and other DGBIs used to be classified as functional GI disorders, or FGIDs. This classification helps to define the difference between GI disorders.

When symptoms include ulcers, blockages (also called obstructions), or a narrowing of the esophagus or intestines (also called strictures), they indicate an issue with the *structure* of the GI tract. When symptoms include bloating, gas, diarrhea, or constipation, they indicate an issue with the *function* of the GI tract. If you have IBS, your doctor will rule out all structural abnormalities first with an endoscopy, colonoscopy, MRI, CT scan, and/or X-ray. Then, they will determine which functional GI disorder you have. Some other tests can diagnose a few functional GI disorders, but unfortunately there is none for IBS to date.

Why Functional GI Disorders are Called Disorders of the Gut–Brain Axis

A long nerve that runs from your brain to your colon is called the vagus nerve. It's your longest cranial nerve and the pathway for signals to run back and forth between our brain and our gut. Have you ever had "butterflies" in your stomach? That anxious feeling might have started in your brain, but your belly is what reacts. Ever feel like you need to poop right after you finish eating even though there is no way that meal made it to the end of your GI tract that quickly? That might be your gut sending mixed signals to your brain. The miscommunication between your gut and your brain is a highlight of irritable bowel syndrome.

Gut microbes play a key role in the connection and disconnect between the gut and the brain in IBS. They produce signaling chemicals called neurotransmitters that can impact brain function. Gut microbes also influence the production of short-chain fatty acids like butyrate, which have anti-inflammatory properties and can positively influence brain function. But when you have an imbalance of the good and the bad microbes, where there are more troublemakers than superheroes, you can get issues like inflammation, barrier dysfunction, and GI symptoms.

Sometimes clients will tell me their IBS stories about when their symptoms started. Many times, they will recall a stomach bug or a bout of food poisoning. The viruses and bacteria that cause these issues can also upset the fine balance of microbes in the gut. As a result, the gut will produce fewer neurotransmitters and SCFAs and disrupt the gut–brain axis. We don't yet fully know the cause of IBS, but research is pointing toward an imbalance of microbes in the microbiome caused by an outside factor.

No matter how IBS starts, it impacts quite a few of us. Approximately 14 percent of the global population is affected by IBS (Arif et al., 2024). The condition is widespread across various regions and demographics, but it seems to be more common in women than in men, with two-thirds of the people who are diagnosed being female. In the U.S., 25–45 million people suffer from IBS, which represents about 8–15 percent of the population. An estimated 11.5 percent of the population in the U.K. has IBS, making it a significant health issue. The prevalence in the U.K. is similar to that in the U.S., with a similar gender disparity.

What Causes IBS?

The short answer: We don't know for sure yet, but researchers are getting closer to naming the cause.

The long answer: The progression of IBS includes a number of issues from all over the body. First is a change in motility (the contracting and mixing movements) of the muscles in the digestive system. They start to function abnormally, slowing down or speeding up the movement of food and waste, which can lead to pain and irregular bowel movements. Second, the gut and the brain have a breakdown in communication across the vagus nerve that runs between your brain and your colon. When the gut–brain axis does not work properly in people with IBS, it can lead to a number of symptoms, including abdominal pain, urgency, bloating, distension, and constipation. All of these issues can cause mental distress, such as anxiety and depression. Believe it or not, emotions play a big role in how your digestive system feels and works. This can create the vicious cycle that can exacerbate symptoms of IBS.

Environmental Factors

Environmental factors can also result in an IBS diagnosis down the road, including early life stressors in childhood such as trauma or difficult experiences. The use of antibiotics, which can disrupt the balance of the microbiome, can be a contributing risk factor, as well as enteric infections like a stomach bug.

Changes in the Immune System

Recent research has also found that changes in the immune system in the gut and the types of microbes in your microbiome might be linked to IBS. Although some of these microbes have been identified, we don't yet have a method for eradicating them, or for changing their balance with respect to other microbes, because we don't know what other functions they may have. That's the cool thing about science: we might not have answers now, but scientists continue to search for answers and hopefully, someday soon, we will have a cure.

Eating Disorders and Disordered Eating

Eating disorders are serious and often fatal mental illnesses that present as severe disturbances in people's eating behaviors and related thoughts and emotions. Some common eating disorders include:

- anorexia nervosa
- bulimia nervosa
- binge eating disorder.

Research shows that over 90 percent of people with eating disorders have functional GI disorders (Janssen, 2010). We don't know the exact mechanism, but the theory is that functional changes along the gut–brain axis are worsened by changes to the microbiome from undernutrition. Malnutrition can also impair the gut's ability to move food and waste, and muscle wasting leads to worse symptoms of constipation, bloating, and abdominal pain.

All of these factors make diagnosing IBS difficult due to the complexity of symptoms and needing to rule out other conditions. In the U.S., it takes approximately six years from the onset of symptoms to be diagnosed. That's a long time of not feeling well! Unfortunately, there is not yet a well-researched biomarker test—like blood, stool, or urine tests as there are for other diseases—so it takes some time to figure out if your symptoms are a sign of IBS or of something else.

How is IBS Diagnosed?

Quite often, I hear people complain that their doctor diagnosed them with IBS when they couldn't come up with any other diagnosis. Although that can feel frustrating, it's not true, but it's also not completely wrong. Irritable bowel syndrome has a set of criteria that need to be met to be properly diagnosed, but many IBS symptoms overlap with those of other GI disorders, so doctors tend to rule them out first. Let's look at the full process.

Rome Wasn't Built in a Day

Criteria for diagnosing IBS were first introduced in the late 1980s when a team of international gastroenterologists formed the Rome Foundation, a non-profit organization. The mission of the Rome Foundation was to develop standardized diagnostic criteria for functional gastrointestinal disorders. They called these Rome I (one) criteria and have updated them every decade or so. We now use Rome IV (four) criteria to diagnose IBS and other DGBIs. This version emphasizes that IBS is a disorder of gut–brain interaction, highlights the role of psychosocial factors and the microbiome, and includes symptom-based criteria.

The symptom-based criteria include recurrent abdominal pain for at least one day a week over the last three months on average and associated with two or more of the following:

1. Moving your bowels.
2. A change in how often you move your bowels.
3. A change in what your bowel movements look like.

These symptoms must have started at least six months before diagnosis. This can feel like a long time to be uncomfortable and without a definitive answer. Still, these criteria and their timeline help your doctor differentiate your symptoms from a stomach virus that may go away in a week or two, or a bout of constipation that may be caused by a new medication or a muscle dysfunction in your pelvic floor unrelated to IBS.

Sound the Alarm!

In addition to the Rome IV criteria, your doctor will rule out what are called *alarm features*. These are symptoms that may indicate a GI disorder that is not IBS but may look like it. Alarm features can include:

- nocturnal diarrhea
- rectal bleeding
- unexplained weight loss of more than 10 percent of your natural body weight over the past three months
- a family history of colorectal cancer, inflammatory bowel disease, or celiac disease.

Your doctor will also complete a physical examination and look for masses in your abdomen and rectum, and will check for swollen or abnormally shaped lymph nodes on your body. They may also check blood work and stool samples for markers of other GI diseases that might look like IBS but are not. Expect a thorough work-up for your diagnosis. Test results may be negative, and you might feel discouraged about not finding a diagnosis and subsequent treatment, but in the long run it's good to get negative results when ruling out alarm features.

Symptoms of IBS

There are a number of general symptoms of IBS that you might experience very differently than another person with IBS. A change in bowel habits is the main criterion for IBS diagnosis, but that can mean different things to different people.

Changes in Bowel Habits

Changes in bowel habits refer not only to how often you are going but also what your poop looks like. There is something called the Bristol Stool Scale that can be used to see where your poop falls (pun intended) from loose to hard.

Soft stool is called diarrhea when it is loose, watery, unformed, and occurs multiple times a day. Stool can be loose and not watery but unformed or in ragged pieces that also occur multiple times a day. These would be a 6 or 7 on the Bristol Stool Scale. It's okay to refer to this as diarrhea too when you speak to your doctor. They might ask you about frequency, texture, and color as well, so sneak a peek in the bowl when you go or take a picture to show them at your next visit. I find that some of my clients with IBS go numerous times in the morning and then maybe once or twice throughout the rest of the day. If you experience this, it's normal for IBS.

Hard stool that is difficult to pass can be a part of constipation. Having incomplete evacuations—feeling like you need to go more but more just won't come out—is also a part of constipation. You may also have a feeling that you have to go but then when you go to the bathroom, nothing passes. This is also a normal experience for people with IBS. Constipation can lead to stool that can look like pebbles or clumps of pebbles. These are a 1 or a 2 on the Bristol Stool Scale.

Keeping track of your Bristol Stool Scale numbers will not only help your gastroenterologist with your IBS diagnosis, it will also help them to determine your subtype. Your IBS subtype allows your doctor and your dietitian to tailor your treatment plan to manage your symptoms.

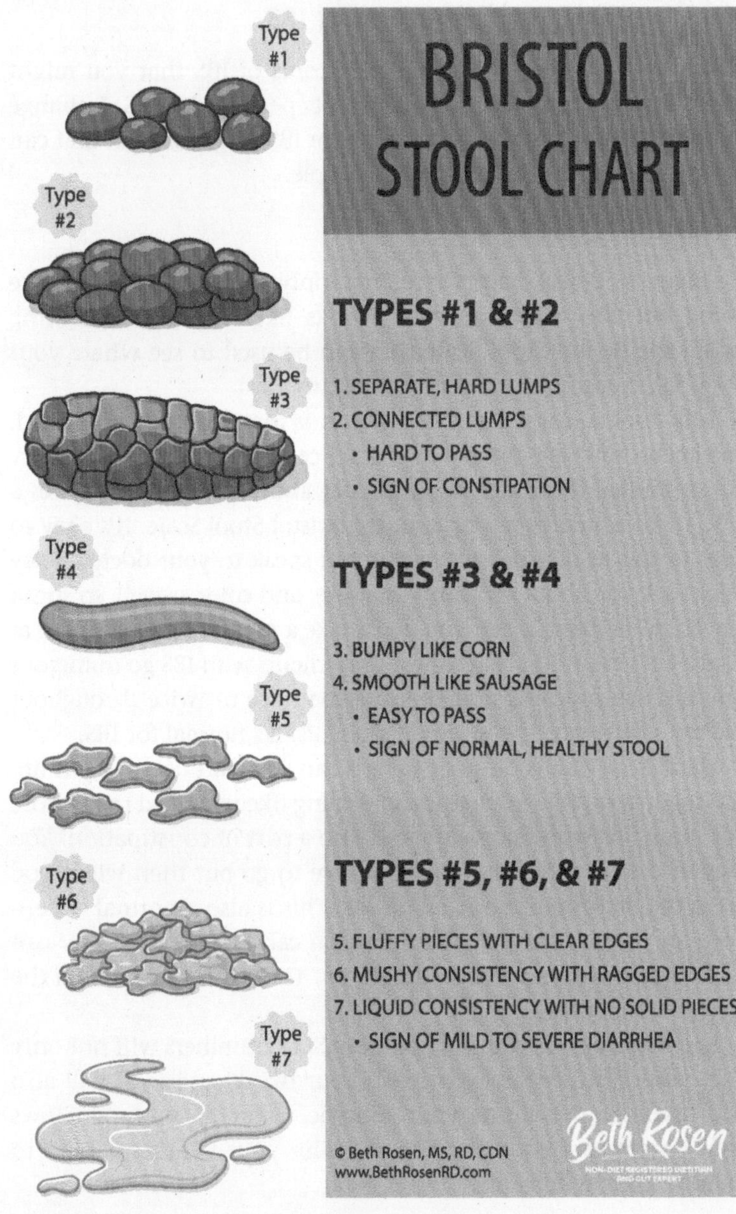

Figure 3.1 The Bristol Stool Scale

Subtypes of IBS

There are four subtypes of IBS and each one is determined by the consistency of your poop and how often you are having stools that are hard or ones that are very soft or watery. Here's the breakdown.

Type	*Description*	*Stool breakdown*
IBS with Constipation (IBS-C)	People who mostly experience constipation	More than 25% of bowel movements are hard or lumpy stools (types 1 and 2 on the Bristol Stool Scale). Less than 25% are loose or watery (types 6 and 7).
IBS with Diarrhea (IBS-D)	People who mostly experience diarrhea	More than 25% of stools are loose or watery (types 6 and 7). Less than 25% are hard or lumpy (types 1 and 2).
IBS with Mixed Bowel Habits (IBS-M)	People who alternate between constipation and diarrhea	More than 25% of stools are hard or lumpy. More than 25% are loose or watery. The pattern can switch back and forth, sometimes even within the same day.
IBS Unsubtyped (IBS-U)	People with inconsistent stool patterns that don't fit into the other categories	Less than 25% of bowel movements are either hard or loose.

Other IBS Symptoms

Diarrhea, constipation, and mixed bowel habits are often accompanied by other symptoms. Not all are universal—people with IBS may have different symptoms but still have the same diagnosis. This is another reason why it can be difficult to diagnose someone with IBS. Some of these symptoms include:

- abdominal discomfort
- gas
- bloating

- distension
- borborygmus
- visceral hypersensitivity.

Abdominal Discomfort

Abdominal discomfort is when your stomach area feels sore, tight, or achy. This feeling can range from mild to excruciating, and it might come and go throughout the day or build as the day goes on. For people with IBS, this discomfort often happens after eating, and it can make you feel uneasy or distracted because your belly just doesn't feel right. Pain is usually not constant and may be alleviated by pooping. It can range from an awareness of having intestines all the way to cramping that disrupts your quality of life.

Gas

Gas is air in your digestive system that needs to escape either through burping or passing gas. When it moves throughout your system or it is trapped, it can cause a feeling of pressure in your abdomen. People with IBS often experience more gas than usual because their digestion works differently, which can make them feel uncomfortable or bloated. Everyone passes gas, whether they have a GI condition or not. The difference is the discomfort associated with it, how often you pass it, and how malodorous it is. The general consensus is that we fart about 15 times a day. Over 25 toots is typically a sign of something gone awry. Smelly gas can be a sign of a change in diet or a new medication, but it can also be a sign of IBS and food intolerances.

Bloating

Bloating is when your belly feels full, tight, or swollen, almost as though it's been pumped up like a balloon. This can happen after you eat or drink something, or just build throughout the day. For people with IBS, bloating can be really bothersome, making clothing, especially waistbands, tight workout pants, and shapewear, feel especially uncomfortable. Bloating is a feeling within the body, but it is not noticeable on the outside of the body.

Distension

Distension is different from bloating and happens when your stomach actually looks larger or puffier than usual. Distension can push out the entire abdomen, but with IBS it typically occurs below the belly button. Some people get distended immediately after eating a meal and some find that the distension builds throughout the day and dissipates overnight. Keep track of when your abdomen becomes distended so that your doctor can use that information to rule out other diagnoses and/or confirm your IBS.

Borborygmus

Borborygmus (bawr-buh-rig-muhs) is perhaps one of my favorite words! It's the word that describes bowel sounds—those funny noises you hear in your gut. Most of the time, that's the sound of gas moving through your intestines. Some people are self-conscious or embarrassed by these sounds, but they are harmless.

Visceral Hypersensitivity

This is perhaps the most frustrating symptom of IBS. Visceral hypersensitivity is an abnormally heightened reaction to a normal amount of stimuli and occurs when there is a miscommunication between the gut and the brain. For instance, you and a friend go out for ice cream and both really enjoy it, but within a few hours your stomach is bloated and distended, you are passing large amounts of gas, and your belly hurts. Your friend is also passing some gas but does not experience any of the other symptoms and seems completely unbothered by the gas. You are experiencing visceral hypersensitivity, or as I often tell my clients: You have a drama queen living in your gut who overreacts to food triggers and other instigators of GI distress. Seriously, visceral hypersensitivity can lead to increased urgency to move your bowels, pain during the digestive process, bloating, and distension. This can become a vicious cycle when anxiety or elevated stress are in the mix, and if your sleep pattern is off or wasn't great to start with.

Visceral hypersensitivity can be exacerbated by intestinal permeability. Remember from Chapter 2 that this permeability occurs between the junctions of the cells of the intestinal lining when those cells that are inflamed are no longer tightly packed together. When particles from within the intestines migrate outside of it, our immune system responds to these foreign bodies and can trigger chronic inflammation outside of the GI tract. This may explain some of the other symptoms of IBS that occur beyond the digestive tract, including fatigue, joint pain, and brain fog. There is some new research showing a correlation between other chronic diseases that begin in the pelvic region of our bodies possibly triggered by the result of intestinal permeability, including endometriosis and interstitial cystitis (Di Vincenzo et al., 2024).

Endometriosis is a condition where tissue that lines the inside of the uterus, called the endometrium, starts growing outside the uterus. This can cause pain, especially during menstrual periods, and may impact fertility. Because the uterus, intestines, and bladder are so tightly packed in the pelvic region, endometrial tissue can connect to these organs and limit their function, and cause pain and IBS symptoms.

Interstitial cystitis is a condition that affects the bladder. The bladder becomes sensitive to being full or empty and mimics the sensation of having to urinate often. It causes pain and discomfort in the bladder and surrounding tissue. It feels similar to a bladder infection, but symptoms do not improve with antibiotics. In my own experience, the *C. diff* infection that caused my IBS and intestinal permeability was most likely the reason for my diagnosis of interstitial cystitis.

While not uncommon for it to occur without IBS, I have seen a number of clients who also have both diagnoses. If you suspect that you might have interstitial cystitis, reach out to your doctor to find a urologist who can help you with a treatment plan. Beware of any restrictive dietary interventions—while there is some correlation between certain foods and symptoms, the causation has not been proven in research. Staying hydrated is most important.

There are a few other symptoms of IBS, but these fall outside of the GI system. They include fatigue, joint pain, and brain fog. Fatigue is more than just being tired. It's a feeling of low energy that doesn't dissipate with rest. People with IBS often have fatigue due to the underlying pain and discomfort that can be draining on your energy stores. We don't know the cause of joint pain in IBS, but it's possible that it is the result of intestinal permeability or the immune system in overdrive. Not all people with IBS will experience joint pain and not all joint pain stems from IBS. Lastly, brain fog describes a feeling of mental confusion or difficulty concentrating. Again, we don't know why this happens, but it may be due to the stress and discomfort from IBS affecting sleep patterns, pain levels, stress, and overall well-being.

What Your Poop Color Means

Stool color	*What it might mean*	*Possible causes*
Brown (normal)	Healthy stool color	Bile from the liver gives poop its normal brown color.
Black or tarry	Possible bleeding in the stomach or small intestine	Ulcers, gastritis, or taking iron supplements or certain medicines (like Pepto-Bismol).
Red	Possible bleeding in the colon, rectum, or anus	Hemorrhoids, small tears (anal fissures), or eating red foods (like beets).
Yellow or green	May indicate digestion or liver problems	Bile duct issues, liver disease, or trouble absorbing fat. Can also happen with diarrhea.
White or clay-colored	Lack of bile	Liver disease, gallbladder issues, or blocked bile ducts.
Orange	Can be caused by diet or medication	Eating foods like carrots or sweet potatoes, or taking certain medicines.
Gray	May indicate liver or pancreas problems	Issues with the liver or pancreas affecting digestion.

Other things to know:

1. Some foods and medications can change stool color temporarily (e.g. red food coloring like in frosting can make it red, iron supplements can make it black).

2. Diarrhea or constipation can also affect stool color.
3. If a color change lasts more than a few days or comes with pain, nausea, or vomiting, let your doctor know.

Now that we have an idea of what IBS is, let's look at all of the possible steps you might take to get a proper diagnosis.

4
Getting a Diagnosis

Neither Dr. Google nor Dr. Reddit will be able to diagnose you with irritable bowel syndrome. Despite what the many people who come to my office with information and misinformation they found on the internet believe, treatment for IBS cannot begin without a proper diagnosis from a gastroenterologist. In Chapter 3, we discussed the need to rule out alarm features when seeking a diagnosis to avoid missing a potentially different disease. If you have something other than IBS, such as celiac disease, ulcerative colitis, or diverticulitis, using the dietary interventions and medications meant for IBS may not be helpful, might be harmful, and will definitely prolong the diagnosis and treatment of whatever else you might have. Living with symptoms of some undiagnosed diseases can lead to a worsening of symptoms and an increased risk and severity of the disease, so seeing your gastroenterologist is essential.

Getting an IBS diagnosis starts with finding a gastroenterologist, who is an expert in all diseases that take place within the GI tract. Some gastroenterologists specialize in different parts of the digestive system like the liver and other accessory organs such as the pancreas, and some have advanced training treating certain diseases like Crohn's disease. Don't worry about finding someone who specializes in IBS—they are all trained to diagnose and treat it.

To find a gastroenterologist, you can check in a few places. If you are in a country where you pay for health insurance, you might check with your insurance company to see who takes your plan so that you have the lowest out-of-pocket expenses. You might also ask for a referral from your primary care doctor. They may have GI doctors that they collaborate with regularly and trust to care for you. Family and friends can share their experiences and recommend a doctor that they like and trust. Lastly, you can use search engines and social media to read reviews of local physicians to find one that feels like a good fit to you.

Once you find a gastroenterologist that you'd like to work with and schedule an appointment, you can prepare by compiling your IBS story.

My IBS Story

When I was on the hunt for answers about why my bowels were behaving the way they were, why I was in pain, and when it would all go away, I found myself starting from square one with every doctor I visited. Instead of spending those precious minutes of my appointment time discussing different treatment options from the ones I had already tried, I was sharing my medical history and medication list, which I had done with every previous doctor. Feeling like a tired old song stuck on repeat, I began to construct a timeline from the first GI symptom to the most recent appointment with the latest doctor to tell me "you're just going to have to learn to live with it." This was the impetus for my IBS story. I brought it with me to every appointment and added new details as they developed. This living document allowed my doctor and me to hit the ground running with what to try next.

Once I had the basics completed, I went back and filled in smaller details that I forgot on my first pass through my IBS journey. In addition to my medical history and medication list, I included the foods I had eliminated, which tools provided relief, and what I had tried but failed to manage my symptoms. When I met with my next (and current) gastroenterologist, I handed him my IBS story. He was both surprised and grateful that I supplied him with all of the information he needed to help me manage my symptoms. I didn't have to go through every medication I had tried and whether or not it worked, and he didn't have to suggest a test that I had already had and which showed nothing of consequence.

He took a few minutes to look through my IBS story. Then he was able to give me a definitive diagnosis and treatment options I had yet to try. This was when he told me that IBS has no cure and would not go away. I appreciated his honesty as he was the first doctor to fully explain this to me. I wept at the prospect of being uncomfortable in my body for the rest of my life, but he assured me that there were many ways to manage symptoms and many more were being researched all over the world. We were able to have these conversations because my IBS story freed up time that would normally be spent during an initial appointment discussing my history and enabled us to use our time together to review options for managing my symptoms.

Your IBS Story

Whether you have IBS symptoms or have had a diagnosis for three months or three years, you can write your own IBS story. It doesn't need to be completed in one sitting if that feels overwhelming. Instead, take it section by section and in a few days you will have a comprehensive document that you can share with your gastroenterologist. I brought mine with me, but that was in the days before there were patient portals and group practice emails. Upload yours to your portal, send it electronically, *and* bring a copy with you. That way, you can ensure that it will be reviewed.

Let's look at some of the sections to include in your IBS story:

- symptoms
- tests
- known/suspected triggers
- medications
- current and past medical history
- healthcare team players.

Symptoms

By now you know that people with IBS have a unique set of symptoms from others who have IBS. When writing your IBS story, include your list of symptoms, a description of how you experience them, and their level of discomfort or severity. For instance, you can list diarrhea as a symptom, but your doctor won't know if that means you have loose stool once a day or if you have urgent, loose stool five or six times a day that is accompanied by abdominal pain and followed by extreme fatigue. Including all of the details, no matter how gross they may seem, will help your doctor know how to best advise you to manage your symptoms.

How often you poop and what your poop looks like, as well as a host of other IBS symptoms, can change from day to day. You may want to keep a symptom log for a week and add that to your story. Be sure to include other, less frequently experienced symptoms you have that may not have occurred during the week you kept a log. Things to include could be the symptoms you experience, how often you are experiencing them, how severe they are (use a scale of 1–5, with 5 being the most severe), how they impact your quality of life (for example, I had to skip class or I needed to find a restroom on my way to work and it made me late), and a section for any thoughts you have on that day. Here's an example of what that might look like.

Tuesday

Symptoms	*Time*	*Severity*	*Quality of life impact*	*Notes*
diarrhea	6:30 am	3	none	First thing in the morning, every day.
diarrhea	7:30 am	3	Running late to work now	
bloating	12:30 pm	1	none	
gas	2:00 pm	4	Really uncomfortable at work	Might have been something I ate at lunch.
diarrhea	4:00 pm	5	So embarrassed about the number of times I go to the bathroom at work each day	Went home right after. Worried that I wouldn't make it home without an accident.
cramping	5:30 pm	2	Had to cancel dinner plans	Stomach feels sore from all of the gas and diarrhea today. Took bismuth subsalicylate and went to bed early.

This sample day may feel extreme to you or it may be what you experience quite often. Your day may include other symptoms, such as:

- constipation
- distension
- nausea
- vomiting
- loss of appetite
- fatigue
- brain fog
- joint pain
- belching
- fear of eating
- increased anxiety.

Even if you have a symptom that doesn't impact your quality of life, it's still important to list it—people with IBS sometimes don't realize that they do not need to live with or get used to the discomfort of this disease if there are tools that can help them reduce or eliminate some or all of their symptoms.

Tests

I want to be very clear about testing: There is no test to definitively diagnose IBS. IBS is diagnosed based on when your symptoms began, and using the criteria of pain and changes in the appearance and frequency of your bowel movements. IBS is also diagnosed by ruling out other diseases, and because of this, your doctor may or may not order testing. There are a number of tests to rule out other diseases and those will be ordered based on your specific symptoms. Because of this, not all people with IBS will have the same tests performed, so don't fret if your list of tests is not the same as someone else's with IBS. For instance, someone with constipation might be tested for a pelvic floor dysfunction (more on that later), while someone with diarrhea might be tested for an enzyme deficiency (more on that below, too). Depending on how long you have been experiencing symptoms, you may have had multiple tests already, or you may not have been tested at all.

It's important to know why you are having tests, so you may want to ask questions. Some things you could consider:

1. What does the test do?
2. What results is my doctor looking for?
3. How should I prepare for the test?
4. When should I expect to hear back about the results?

Some tests are quick, like going for blood work, while others may take a day or two of preparation by changing your diet or temporarily stopping medication. Having all of the information about tests ensures that you are properly prepared and won't be turned away and need to reschedule because you did something wrong. To help you prepare, here are some of the tests that you might encounter.

Blood Tests

Your blood holds lots of information about what's going on in your body. Blood tests can be quick and easy (as long as you don't mind needles). When you go to a lab to have your blood drawn, the technician will either ask for the requisition from your doctor or ask for your information to find it in their computer system. Once they have confirmed what tests were ordered, they will draw blood from your arm or a vein in the back of your hand into vials that get sent to a lab. If you have a portal with your doctor's office, your lab results will be posted there. Some results come back quickly; these are usually the tests that measure the amount of something in your blood. Some tests take longer because they are watching to see if something is growing (called a culture). Some blood tests that may be ordered include those to rule out infection and the genes for celiac disease.

Here are some of the tests you might see listed on your lab requisite:

1. HLA DQ2 and HLA DQ8: These are the genes for celiac disease. Someone who has these genes is at risk of having or getting celiac disease, but if you do not have the genes, you will never get celiac disease. This gene test is not a diagnosis for celiac disease, but if you do have the genes, it indicates that you are

at an increased risk and should speak to your doctor about next steps.

2. Tissue transglutaminase (tTg-IgA): This test looks for antibodies or immune cells that are present in people with celiac disease as a sign that the body is reacting negatively to the presence of gluten in the diet. It is usually the first test done to rule out celiac disease but might be done at the same time as the gene test.
3. C-reactive protein: This protein is produced by the liver and is present when there is inflammation in the body. It is not specific to GI diseases but may be a sign that there is something amiss in your body and may lead to further testing.
4. Erythrocyte sedimentation rate: This test looks at how quickly red blood cells settle at the bottom of a test tube. The quicker they settle, the more likely it is that there is inflammation and swelling in your body. This test is not a diagnostic tool but it provides data for your doctor to decide what other tests might be needed.
5. Complete blood count (CBC): Most likely you've had this test numerous times in your life. This test looks at a number of types of cells in your blood, including white blood cells. When white blood cell measurements are not within a normal range, it can be an indication of infection.

Stool Tests

Because IBS doesn't show up in any specific test, doctors may order stool tests to check for signs of inflammation, infection, or other digestive conditions. By using these tests, they can make sure that symptoms aren't being caused by conditions such as inflammatory bowel disease (IBD)—Crohn's and ulcerative colitis—or problems with the pancreas or gallbladder.

Stool tests are ... gross. They come with a shallow cover, which you place over your toilet seat, and you poop into it. Depending on what test you are having done, you may have containers to fill that are empty or that have a solution in them. You will scoop stool into the containers, close them, and then get them to the lab as soon as possible. If you can't get to the lab quickly, some containers can be refrigerated while some can be frozen. Make sure to ask if this is something you can do if you can't drop them off right away. Most samples have to be brought to the lab within hours of collection.

Here are some of the stool tests you might encounter:

1. Fecal calprotectin: This test checks for inflammation in the intestines. Calprotectin is a protein found in white blood cells, and when there's inflammation, more of this protein is released into the stool. High levels may suggest inflammatory bowel disease, which your doctor needs to rule out before diagnosing IBS.
2. Fecal lactoferrin: Lactoferrin is another protein found in white blood cells. Like calprotectin, increased levels of lactoferrin in stool point to inflammation in the gut. This helps doctors distinguish between IBS, which doesn't trigger inflammatory markers, and IBD, which does.
3. Fecal elastase: This test measures elastase, an enzyme produced by the pancreas. Low levels can signal issues with the pancreas, which may cause symptoms similar to IBS. This helps to rule out pancreatic diseases like exocrine pancreatic insufficiency as the cause of digestive symptoms.
4. Parasites: This test checks for organisms that can live in the digestive system and cause infections. A stool sample can help find parasites like Giardia which can cause diarrhea and mimic symptoms of IBS.
5. Bacterial infections: Testing for bacterial infections in the gut is necessary because they can lead to symptoms like diarrhea and cramping that might be temporary, unlike IBS. *C. difficile*, the bacterial infection I had, was found in a stool test. *E. coli*, which can be caused by food poisoning, is another bacterial infection that can present as IBS symptoms but can be treated with antibiotics and go away.
6. Fecal bile acid excretion: Bile acids help digest fats, but sometimes they aren't absorbed well and can irritate the intestines, causing diarrhea. This is called bile acid malabsorption or bile acid diarrhea. While it may have symptoms similar to IBS, some telling signs are in the toilet—floating stool or an

oily appearance to the water in the bowl after pooping may indicate that fat is not being absorbed. The good news is that there is medication for bile acid malabsorption.

Breath Tests

Breath tests are another tool doctors use when ruling out other diagnoses, especially when symptoms might be caused by the way the body processes certain sugars, or by an overgrowth of the "bad" bugs in the gut.

Breath tests work by measuring gases like hydrogen and methane in the breath, which are produced when bacteria in the intestines break down food. When specific foods or carbohydrates aren't digested properly, these gases increase and are detected in the breath test. This helps doctors identify issues like small intestinal bacterial overgrowth, lactose intolerance, and sucrase-isomaltase deficiency.

Small Intestinal Bacterial Overgrowth (SIBO) SIBO occurs when too many microbes grow in the small intestine, where they don't usually live.

Shared SIBO and IBS symptoms:

- gas
- constipation
- diarrhea
- bloating.

While SIBO and IBS have many similar symptoms, one possible difference is where bloating and distension occur. People with IBS tend to feel bloating in the lower abdomen while those with SIBO feel it in the upper abdomen. Some of my clients have reported pressure in their chest, under their ribs, and above their belly button. I use this clue to refer them back to their gastroenterologist for SIBO testing. It's not uncommon, though, for people to have SIBO *and* IBS. In fact, there has been research suggesting that 60 percent of people with SIBO also have IBS (Takakura and Pimentel, 2020). If you have upper abdominal bloating in addition to your IBS symptoms, you might have SIBO.

The SIBO test measures hydrogen and methane gas levels in your breath. High levels of these gases suggest that microbes are fermenting the sugars in the small intestine, which could be causing symptoms. This test can be done in a doctor's office, but there are also at-home test kits available. You will have to prepare for the test by altering your diet the day before and putting some of your medications and supplements on pause for up to a month before, especially antibiotics and probiotics.

The test will come with a sugary solution. You'll drink the solution and then blow into a tube connected to a small, inflatable bag. You will be asked to blow into a tube every 15–20 minutes for a few hours. In between, you will sit in the office and wait. If you take the at-home test, you will have to set a timer so that you can make the breath collections on time. If you are being tested in a doctor's office, the results will be shared with you when the test is over. For the at-home test, you will need to wait for about a week for the lab to process your results and send you a report.

The results for hydrogen-predominant SIBO are measured in parts per million (ppm). If your hydrogen gas level goes to 20 ppm or more in the first 90 minutes, then you have a positive SIBO test (not positive as in, "Oh that's awesome!" but positive in that you have it). You can also have a positive SIBO test if your methane colony count measures above the cutoff number of 10^3 at any time during the test. No test is perfect and there can be some false positive results. These can be due to testing errors or lab errors. To ensure that your test results are not at risk of a false positive, make sure to follow all pre-test requirements for diet, medication, and test kit use.

The silver lining is that unlike IBS, SIBO can be cured. There are antibiotics that are specifically designed to target SIBO and kill off the overgrowth. The downside is that the antibiotics don't always work on the first try, but they are safe enough to take up to three rounds over six months. Your doctor can prescribe them for you once you have a diagnosis. You might find some people on the internet selling antimicrobial supplements to help eradicate SIBO, or purporting their benefits, but there is currently no scientific research supporting the claims.

Lactose Intolerance Lactose intolerance happens when the body can't break down lactose, the naturally occurring sugar in milk. This is because of a lack of lactase, an enzyme needed to digest lactose. Lactose is typically produced in the small intestine, but many people stop making enough due to genetics or illness that can damage the cells that produce lactose.

Shared lactose intolerance and IBS symptoms:

- diarrhea
- constipation
- gas
- bloating.

The breath test can detect if the carbohydrate component in dairy is the cause of your symptoms. During the test, you will drink a lactose-containing solution. If the lactose is not digested by the body's enzymes, then the lactose will move into the small intestine and be fermented by microbes. This produces hydrogen gas, which will show up in your breath.

The silver lining is that there are over-the-counter forms of lactase that you can take with your meals that contain dairy products. The dose is 9,000 units (usually 1–3 pills depending on the brand you buy) and it will last 30 minutes when taken with your first bite. Digestive enzymes like lactase are proteins so they are perfectly safe for you to take multiple times per day. What your body doesn't use for lactose, it will digest as safely as it does protein.

Lactose intolerance, while uncomfortable when you don't take the digestive enzyme, leads to IBS-like symptoms, but is otherwise harmless. People with celiac disease tend to be prone to lactose intolerance due to the damage that gluten does to the part of the small intestine that produces lactase. It's important to rule out celiac disease if your doctor suspects IBS, so you might be asked about your eating patterns in relation to your symptoms and sent for blood work.

Sucrase-Isomaltase Deficiency Sucrase-isomaltase deficiency (SID) is a condition where the body can't digest certain sugars, like sucrose (table sugar) and starches.

Shared SID and IBS symptoms:

- gas
- cramping
- bloating
- diarrhea.

Please note, all these symptoms only show up after eating some sweet or starchy foods, unlike with IBS.

One of the biggest differences between IBS and sucrase-isomaltase deficiency that I have seen among my clients is that those who have bloating as an IBS symptom tend to wake up in the morning without bloat, while those with SID wake up without relief from bloating even after an overnight fast and sleep.

The breath test for this deficiency measures hydrogen levels after consuming a solution with these sugars. The abnormal ranges for sucrase enzyme activity for men are less than 3.9 percent and for women are less than 5.2 percent. If your numbers are lower, then you will be prescribed an enzyme to help digest sucrose. Currently, there is no enzyme supplement on the market that breaks down starches. It is possible to test positive and only have symptoms after eating sucrose and not starch. Working with a registered dietitian to determine if you tolerate starches, and what your tolerance level is per meal and snack, will help you to manage your symptoms and liberalize your diet.

Just like other breath tests, the sucrose breath test is not always accurate. The most accurate test for SID is called a sucrase assay via endoscopy. This test takes a sample of your small intestine and tests it for enzyme activity. It is the gold standard for diagnosing SID, but it is also quite expensive and not readily available to patients due to few labs that test for sucrase activity in the world.

Other Tests

Endoscopy Endoscopy is a medical procedure that helps doctors look inside your digestive system using a thin, flexible tube with a camera and a light at the end. This tool, called an endoscope, allows them to examine areas like your esophagus, stomach, and small intestine to uncover what might be causing your symptoms.

While endoscopy isn't used to directly diagnose IBS, it plays an essential role in ruling out other conditions that can mimic IBS symptoms.

Some of the issues that can be diagnosed using endoscopy are lactose intolerance, SIBO, and SID, but there are others. Here are a few that your doctor may look for in their quest to diagnose you with IBS and rule out other issues.

Eosinophilic Esophagitis (EoE) EoE is a condition where a type of white blood cell called eosinophils builds up in the esophagus, often due to an allergic reaction. It can cause symptoms such as trouble swallowing or feeling like food is stuck in your throat or chest. During an endoscopy, the doctor can look for signs of inflammation or narrowing in the esophagus and take samples of the esophagus to check for the presence of eosinophils. If they diagnose you with EoE, treatments like diet changes and medications can help.

***Helicobacter Pylori* Infection (*H. pylori*)** *H. pylori* is a type of bacteria that can live in the stomach and cause problems like ulcers, bloating, or stomach pain. For some, it can feel like heartburn or indigestion. During an endoscopy, doctors can collect a sample of the stomach lining to test for this. There are other tests for *H. pylori* such as blood and stool collection, but the biopsy via endoscopy is the most accurate.

Shared *H. pylori* and IBS symptoms:

- bloating
- stomach pain.

Celiac Disease Celiac disease is an autoimmune condition where eating gluten, a protein found in wheat, barley, and rye, damages the lining of the small intestine. Endoscopy allows doctors to take biopsies from the small intestine to look for this damage.

Shared celiac disease and IBS symptoms:

- diarrhea
- constipation
- bloating

- abdominal pain
- fatigue
- joint pain.

The only treatment for celiac disease currently is a strict gluten-free diet. If left untreated, or if gluten-containing foods are consumed, it can lead to issues from vitamin deficiencies to cancer. It is possible to have both IBS and celiac disease, but it is also important to rule it out because the symptoms might be similar.

Colonoscopy A colonoscopy is a procedure that lets your doctor look inside your colon (aka large intestine) using a long, flexible tube with a camera and a light at the end. A colonoscopy requires preparation. The day before, you'll need to consume only clear foods and liquids (thick broth, gelatin), late in the day you'll drink a solution that will completely empty your bowels, and then you'll fast to clear the colon so that the lining can be seen and biopsied.

If you have IBS and no other disease of the colon, you will most likely be informed by your doctor that your colonoscopy was "clear" or "unremarkable." This can feel dismissive or disappointing, especially if the information is delivered as such, but it's important to keep in mind that IBS is a *functional* disease and not a *structural* disease. Remember that this means that the appearance of your colon is good—no ulcers, narrowing, or damaged bits—but a colonoscopy can't measure how well your large intestine works. The use of the colonoscopy for IBS is to rule out the diseases that lead to ulcers, narrowing, and damaged bits. It may be hard to do, but consider a "clear" or "unremarkable" colonoscopy report to be a silver lining in your GI journey.

The following are some of the diseases that your doctor will be looking to rule out during your colonoscopy.

Crohn's Disease Crohn's disease is a type of inflammatory bowel disease that can affect any part of the digestive tract, including the colon.

Shared Crohn's disease and IBS symptoms:

- diarrhea
- abdominal pain.

A colonoscopy can reveal inflammation, ulcers, or damage to the colon. Biopsies might also be taken to confirm the diagnosis. It is possible to have IBS and Crohn's disease, but they require different treatment plans. Controlling inflammation and preventing complications is essential to managing Crohn's disease and minimizing progression.

Ulcerative Colitis (UC) UC is another type of IBD, but it only affects the colon and rectum. It causes inflammation and ulcers in the lining of the colon. Unlike with IBS, one of the symptoms of UC is diarrhea with blood and/or mucus present. This is an alarm feature that you should bring up with your doctor.

Shared UC and IBS symptoms:

- abdominal pain
- urgency to use the bathroom.

Like Crohn's, a biopsy will be taken to confirm the disease. Also like Crohn's, it is possible to have both UC and IBS, but the treatment plan is different, so getting that diagnosis is integral to obtaining proper treatment and minimizing flares.

Diverticular Diseases Diverticulosis happens when small pouches, called diverticula, form in the colon wall. Diverticula are common and don't cause symptoms. Diverticulitis, however, happens when the diverticula become inflamed or infected. A telling symptom is a fever, along with symptoms that feel like IBS.

Shared diverticulitis and IBS symptoms:

- diarrhea
- abdominal pain.

A colonoscopy can confirm the presence of diverticulosis so that you can take steps to reduce the chances of developing diverticulitis.

Colon Polyps or Cancer Colon polyps are small growths on the lining of the colon and don't usually cause symptoms. During a colonoscopy, your doctor will remove polyps and biopsy them to check for cancer cells. While small polyps don't usually cause symptoms, larger polyps and those that develop into colon cancer can lead to bleeding and symptoms that look a lot like IBS.

Shared colon polyps and IBS symptoms:

- changes in bowel habits
- abdominal pain.

Many, many GI diseases have similar symptoms and it's important to share them all with your doctor so that they can catch problems early.

Microscopic Colitis Microscopic colitis is a condition in which the colon looks normal during a colonoscopy, but under a microscope in biopsy samples the lab can detect tiny inflammation. Microscopic colitis can cause watery diarrhea and other symptoms similar to IBS but requires a different treatment.

Shared microscopic colitis and IBS symptoms:

- diarrhea
- abdominal pain
- distension.

By the way, I am not the only one in my family with a GI condition—my husband was diagnosed with microscopic colitis a few years after I was diagnosed with IBS. Fortunately, he was able to see my wonderful gastroenterologist and he has been flare-free for years.

If you have been scheduled for a colonoscopy, know that it is a powerful tool for ruling out other diseases and giving you information you need to understand your IBS. As gross and as scary as it may seem to you, it's an important information-gathering procedure that will bring you a step closer to an IBS diagnosis and confirm that there is nothing structurally wrong with your large intestine.

CT Scan A CT scan is a helpful tool in the diagnostic process as it provides a clear picture of what's happening inside your body.

It allows your doctor to quickly rule out serious conditions that might be causing your symptoms. If the scan shows no signs of these issues, it helps confirm an IBS diagnosis and guides the next steps for managing your symptoms.

A CT scan can see lots of things inside your body, but it has some limits. When looking for GI-related conditions, your doctor will be able to see organs such as the liver, kidneys, pancreas, and intestines, and whether there is inflammation or masses in these tissues. A CT scan can also show blood vessels, abscesses, tumors, diverticulitis, appendicitis, and stones in the gallbladder. It can provide good overall detail but cannot show functionality or microscopic abnormalities, so CT scans are often used alongside other tests like ultrasounds, endoscopies, and colonoscopies.

X-ray An X-ray uses low levels of radiation to create images of your body. In digestive health, X-rays are often used to check for problems like blockages, constipation, or abnormal shapes in the colon. It's quick and easy to have an X-ray but it doesn't test for *functionality* (notice a pattern with all of these tests thus far?).

Anal Manometry Anal manometry measures the strength and coordination of the muscles in your rectum and anus. During this test, a small tube with a balloon is inserted into the rectum to measure muscle pressure as you relax, squeeze, and push. This test can feel embarrassing, but it is quick and will give your doctor information about the function of your anus and rectum to help you properly empty your bowels.

Defecography Defecography is a specialized imaging test that examines how the rectum and pelvic floor function during a bowel movement. The test involves inserting a soft paste (similar to stool) into the rectum, and X-rays or MRI images are then taken as you attempt to pass it. This test can feel mortifying because you are pooping (even if it's not real poop) in front of medical professionals, but it provides a clear picture of how the rectum and pelvic floor muscles work together (or don't) when you poop, and can identify issues like muscle coordination problems and pelvic organ dysfunction and thus allow for treatment of those issues.

Pelvic Floor Evaluations Pelvic floor evaluations assess how well the muscles in your pelvic area work together. These muscles support the bladder, uterus (if you have one), and rectum, and help with bowel movements. Evaluations may include physical exams, imaging, or defecography. If you do have a pelvic floor dysfunction, you will be referred to a pelvic floor physical therapist who will help you retrain those muscles and get your system working properly again.

Tests to Avoid

There are so many people with GI issues that it has made for an enormous money-making opportunity for the medical industrial complex. This is not to say that there aren't some "good guys" out there looking to help you feel better. Unfortunately, when a trend emerges like more people receiving GI-related diagnoses, you can bet that there are some not-so-good guys bringing products to the market that have not gone through rigorous testing or randomized controlled trials to guarantee that they work and have valid results. The companies that have developed these products have marketing masterminds at work, so it is rare that they will readily provide information on whether or not their product has been tested, how it's been tested, and the results of those tests.

While some of these tools are great in theory, many times they fall short in reality. Here are a few that are currently available but should not be used.

IgG Antibody Food Sensitivity Testing IgG tests measure antibodies in your blood that supposedly show how your immune system reacts to certain foods. The idea is that high levels of IgG antibodies mean you're intolerant or sensitive to those foods and avoiding them will improve your symptoms. IgG antibodies are "memory" antibodies—they will be able to tell whether that food has been in your system before—but what they can't do is tell whether you had an adverse reaction to that food.

These tests often list dozens of foods to be avoided, which can lead to unnecessary restriction and food fear. There is enough research to show that these tests are not reliable for diagnosing food intolerances, allergies, or sensitivities.

Lifestyle Eating and Performance (LEAP) and Mediator Release Test (MRT) Testing LEAP and MRT purport to analyze your body's reaction to different foods and chemicals in a test tube that combines your blood and the food/chemical. These tests lack scientific validation. The methods used to identify food sensitivities aren't proven to be accurate, and like IgG food sensitivity testing, the diet plans created from these results often eliminate foods unnecessarily.

Microbiome Mapping Microbiome mapping tests analyze the bacteria and other microorganisms in your gut. They promise to provide detailed insights into your gut health by giving measurements of the amounts of various microbes and pathogens that might be present. The biggest issue with testing the microbiome is that we do not yet have enough data to know what a "healthy" microbiome should consist of, or to know that we have identified all of the microbes that might inhabit our gut. In theory, this is a really insightful test, but in reality it goes beyond what is known in current science. Taking this test will not give you answers about your gut health, but it will empty your pockets of some money because the test is not covered by health insurers.

Known and Suspected Triggers

As you continue to write your IBS story, you will want to include your known and suspected triggers for symptoms. You may have a very clear idea of what sets off GI distress and may have minimized or reduced those triggers, and yet you still have symptoms. Your known triggers might be accurate, but there might be others you haven't identified yet. Make sure to include all of your thoughts about what might be exacerbating your discomfort. In the next chapter, we will go through possible triggers in depth.

Medications

Keeping an updated list of all of the medications you take is an important piece of your story. You will want to include what you are currently taking, who prescribed the medication, the reason for the medication, and the dosage. Your list should include any over-the-counter medication, vitamins, supplements, and herbal products that you take regularly as well as any prescribed or over-the counter medications that you take only when needed. For instance, if you take a multivitamin, a medication for high blood pressure, and baby aspirin daily, list those. If you take an anti-inflammatory medication only when your knee hurts, list that too. Your doctor will want to check for any drug–drug interactions that may be detrimental to your health, but also see if any of your medications have gastrointestinal-related side effects.

I had a new client come to me with long-standing IBS who was recently diagnosed with gastroparesis (delayed stomach emptying). She provided her medication list and I noticed that one of the medications for a mental health diagnosis was one that is known to slow gastric emptying. She was asked to share any side effects with her prescriber, but because she was experiencing GI distress, she assumed the two were not related and didn't report it. I referred her back to her prescriber who changed her medication and within a matter of days she felt relief.

Create your list and keep it with you—either on your phone or in your wallet—and make sure to update it regularly. We are asked so many questions at healthcare visits that we are bound to forget something. Don't let that something be what medications you are taking—it could make finding solutions to your IBS issues quicker.

Current and Past Medical History and Your Healthcare Team

In a perfect world, all of your physicians, dietitians, and healthcare providers would have access to everything about your health, review it before meeting with you, consult with each other about possible solutions, and then share their thoughts with you on possible options for care. Because this perfect world does not exist, you will have to be the point person. You will want to share what other diagnoses you are currently being treated for, who is treating you, and their contact information (in case collaboration is in the cards). You will also want to list what you have been treated for in the past. This may include past cancer diagnoses, kidney infections, and surgeries, to name a few.

Getting a diagnosis for IBS can be a long journey. You may start with one symptom and then find that others evolve along the way. Everybody's IBS diagnosis is different and your IBS story is uniquely yours, shaped by your experiences, symptoms, and the path you've taken to find answers. Getting to a diagnosis requires patience and persistence. By documenting your symptoms, suspected triggers, medical history, medications, and diagnostic tests, you create a comprehensive resource that empowers both you and your healthcare team, so get started!

5
Triggers—The Triumvirate

It's so easy to blame food when it comes to experiencing IBS symptoms. What goes into our body must be the cause of what happens inside of it, right? Well, partially right.

After my *C. diff* infection and subsequent IBS diagnosis, I was still experiencing symptoms quite often. I, too, assumed that my triggers were food-related. Every time I experienced a symptom, I would recall my most recent meal, find a food that could possibly be the culprit, and remove it from my diet. This continued over a few months and what I found was that while my diet became more restricted and less varied, my symptoms did not drastically improve, and I was left with little food to choose from and still experiencing daily discomfort. I know that I am not alone in this practice of:

- removing food
- not having symptom relief
- not introducing the food that was wrongly accused back into my diet.

I've had numerous clients come to me with a list of foods they have been eating that could be counted on one to two hands and not connect the dots that the symptoms were not alleviated by the food elimination.

If this sounds familiar, you are in good but misguided company. Yes, food can be a trigger for IBS symptoms. It does make sense that what goes into the body can impact it. But it's not the only possible cause of your symptoms. There are two other main causes of IBS symptoms that complete the triumvirate: stress and sleep.

Understanding these triggers is a crucial step in managing IBS effectively. Your experience with IBS is unique, and by identifying specific factors that exacerbate your symptoms, you can use targeted strategies and make informed choices to reduce the frequency, duration, and intensity of flares. The ultimate goal of identifying your trigger or triggers is improved quality of life. Let's look at food, stress, and sleep and see the role they might play in your digestive discomfort.

Food

There are three ways in which food can trigger IBS symptoms. The first is its impact on the gut–brain interaction, the second is the way they are acted upon by our microbiome, and the third is how a food intolerance or food allergy can provoke a cascade effect resulting in symptoms.

In Chapter 2 we discussed the function of the gut–brain axis, the two-way communication system that connects your digestive system and your brain. This system plays a significant role in IBS and is the reason why food is one of the biggest triggers. The job of the brain in this axis is to send signals to your gut to carry out digestive tasks. These can include regulating how quickly food moves through your system, how much digestive juices and enzymes are released, and how sensitive you will be to the sensations that occur during digestion. The gut's job is to send information back to the brain, such as when you are hungry, when you've reached fullness, and when you experience GI discomfort.

As you may recall, this communication system doesn't always function smoothly in people with IBS. The gut may overreact to normal digestive processes, leading to pain, bloating, or diarrhea. Certain foods may set off this overreaction, not because they're inherently "bad" but because the gut–brain axis misinterprets them as a problem. Remember I mentioned that there is a drama queen living in your gut? Here she is.

One of the key players in this process is the gut's microbiome—the trillions of microbes that live in your digestive tract. These organisms that help break down food, support your immune system, and even affect your mood can increase gut sensitivity when out of balance and lead to IBS symptoms. Food for thought: Maybe instead of one drama queen, you've got trillions!

The third way that food can lead to IBS symptoms is due to an intolerance or an allergy to that food. Food intolerance and food allergy are different, although the terms are sometimes used interchangeably. If you have a food allergy, your body will react to that food with an immune response—your immune system detects the food as a harmful substance and sets off a chemical reaction that is supposed to protect you from harm but instead leads to allergy symptoms. These symptoms can include everything from itchiness and hives to anaphylaxis, an inability to breathe that can possibly result in death if left untreated. Food intolerances, meanwhile, do not set off the immune response but can lead to GI upset and IBS symptoms that are not life-threatening. If you suspect you have a food allergy, it's important that you get tested by a specialist so that you can take the proper precautions to keep yourself safe. If you think you might have a food intolerance, then working with a registered dietitian to confirm it and find nutritionally equivalent food substitutes will make for fewer IBS flares.

Types of Food That Can Be Triggers

I've seen clients remove all types of foods from their diets, from brand-specific raw chicken to cereal that contained an additive that turned out to be a vitamin. If you spend time on the internet, chances are you will find others doing the same. Although it may seem that all foods can trigger symptoms, it is highly unlikely. However, there is strong evidence from years of research indicating that foods that contain *fermentable carbohydrates* are more likely to contribute to GI distress in people with IBS.

Fermentable carbohydrates are specific fibers, sugars, and starches that are not digested by the body. This is because they either can't be broken down due to a missing enzyme or they are naturally indigestible. When these foods are consumed, microbes feed off them and produce gas, or the carbohydrate is not broken down earlier in the digestion process and ends up as a bigger molecule in the large intestine where it will draw in water and cause bloating and/or loose stools. People without IBS eat these foods every day without thought or consequence, but because of visceral hypersensitivity (aka the drama queen), people with IBS will experience gas, bloating, abdominal cramping, and other symptoms from ingestion of foods that contain fermentable carbohydrates that are their trigger foods.

Not all fermentable carbohydrates will trigger symptoms in people with IBS, even if food is a trigger. There are a few categories of these carbohydrates that we will explore more deeply in the next chapter, but examples of common fermentable carbohydrates in food include:

- wheat
- milk
- mushrooms
- apples
- lentils
- garlic.

As you can see from these examples, fermentable carbohydrates contain lots of nutrients that would otherwise be included in a "healthy" diet. I put healthy in quotes because the term is subjective. If you ate a diet rich in fiber-filled foods as recommended by health professionals and you have IBS, it's possible that you would feel your *unhealthiest* after consuming them. A healthy diet is one where you thrive, have energy, and reduce health risks. If someone with IBS were to consume fermentable carbohydrates that triggered their symptoms, thriving would probably be the last word they would use to describe themselves.

For those without IBS (and those with IBS who can tolerate them), fermentable carbohydrates offer wonderful health benefits. They are prebiotics—food for the gut microbes—and help to maintain balance in the microbiome. Fiber from these foods helps regulate digestion, blood glucose, and bowel habits. The goal, then, for people with IBS is to figure out that if food is a trigger for symptoms, which food or foods are causing the issue and only eliminate those from the diet. In the next chapter, we will talk in depth on how to do just that.

Beyond fermentable carbohydrates, there are some foods that can irritate the GI tract and increase or exacerbate symptoms. Caffeine, found in coffee, tea, and some sodas, is a stimulant and can quicken the pace of digestion by stimulating the muscles in the gut to work faster. This can lead to diarrhea and urgency to move your bowels.

Carbonated beverages like soda, seltzer, and sparkling water can also impact digestion negatively for some. Those bubbly beverages contain gas, and when ingested, that gas enters the GI tract. Some people are not bothered by it, yet some feel increased pressure in their stomach, have more belching, reflux, and bloating after consumption. If you are among them, you might consider bubble-free beverages.

Alcohol and spices can also trigger symptoms by irritating the gut lining, leading to an overproduction of mucus and making stools very soft. Beer and sparkling drinks like prosecco and champagne are carbonated and have double the chance of irritating the gut beyond wine and spirits. Spicy food can also lead to GI pain for some. The good news is that all herbs are neither fermentable carbohydrates nor contain any ingredient known to cause GI distress in those with IBS and that leaves many options for seasoning your food without pain or discomfort.

Stress

It would make sense that the gut–brain axis with the vagus nerve at the helm—that nerve that runs from the brain to the colon—can be impacted by stress. When we experience stress, our body sets off the fight-or-flight response. This is a reaction that lives deep within our brain and has been instinctual since our caveman days. It has kept us safe from predators for millions of years. Much of how our brain functions has evolved in the millennia since, but the fight-or-flight response remains—it will activate every time we sense danger and is not nuanced enough to know the difference between true and perceived danger. How I explain this to my clients is that their fight-or-flight response doesn't know the difference between the fear of being chased by a saber-tooth tiger and the fear of a stomachache from eating an apple. In both instances, the result leads to changes in how our digestive tract functions.

Imagine for a moment that you are being chased by that tiger. You would need every bit of energy in your body to go to your legs to run and your arms to pump to get you to move as fast as you could. Your body helps you with this by releasing two hormones, cortisol and adrenaline, and giving you a burst of energy to get the heck out of danger. While you are running, blood is diverted away from your GI tract and into your extremities. This slows your digestion while your body prioritizes running to safety. Even though you aren't technically running from the apple, your caveman brain doesn't know the difference and the same cascade of events occurs. When blood is diverted away from the digestive tract, digestion slows, food that is in the tract can be fermented by the microbes, gas can build up, bloating can develop, and constipation can begin.

Slowed digestion is one way that stress can impact the GI tract. Heightened stress can also cause an increase in visceral hypersensitivity. That drama queen loves stress and she will boost pain signals at the first sign of it, cause constipation, or speed up gut transit time and signal to empty in moments of stress. If you've ever needed to move your bowels right before going on stage or before a big game, you've got the fight-or-flight stress response to thank.

The gut microbiome does not come away from stress unscathed. Stress can lead to an imbalance of microbes by reducing the beneficial ones and allowing the growth of the harmful bugs. Stress worsens IBS symptoms, and the symptoms themselves create more stress and anxiety. This vicious cycle is hard to slow down.

Types of Stress

There are a few types of stress that can impact your IBS symptoms. Knowing which one you are experiencing can help you to determine how best to manage it (we will get to management tools in Chapter 7). Three main types include:

- specific stressful events
- ongoing life challenges
- emotional states or mental health diagnoses.

Specific stressful events, or acute stress, arise from short-term, specific situations such as a work deadline, public speaking, or a sudden conflict (like being chased by a saber-tooth tiger). For people with IBS, even brief stressors can trigger flare-ups, leading to symptoms. Even though the stressor is temporary, its impact can last from a few hours to a few days.

Ongoing life challenges, or chronic stress, can come from responsibilities at home or at work, financial struggles, or caregiving. In these cases, the body is in a prolonged state of stress. This type of stress is constant and can cause persistent symptoms and inflammation in the gut, leading to flares that are longer and more painful.

Emotional states like anxiety and depression are closely linked to IBS through the gut–brain axis. Anxiety can heighten gut sensitivity, making even minor digestive disturbances feel severe. Serotonin, a neurotransmitter that regulates mood and GI motility, is made in the gut. Depression, which is associated with low serotonin levels, can disrupt both emotional well-being and digestive function. Anxiety and depression can make it harder to manage acute and chronic stress, as well as managing living with a chronic disease like IBS, creating another vicious cycle where IBS symptoms and emotional struggles set off one another.

Sleep

Sleep and IBS symptoms don't seem as though they could be connected, but you'd be surprised how much of a role our circadian rhythm—the internal clock responsible for sleeping and waking, hormone release, immune response, and yes, digestion—plays in triggering IBS symptoms. It makes sense, then, that poor sleep can leave you feeling tired but can also worsen symptoms and form yet *another* vicious cycle—poor sleep leads to worse IBS symptoms, and those symptoms make it harder to sleep.

When you sleep, your body goes into repair mode, giving your digestive system time to rest and reset. You might find that you fall asleep feeling bloated but wake up without any pressure or negative sensation in your belly. During this repair period, sleep also helps in regulating the gut–brain axis by allowing the vagus nerve to reset, regulating the hormones that are released when you are stressed, and indirectly impacting the immune system that plays a role in gut inflammation and pain signals. Poor sleep disrupts this balance. Studies show that people with IBS who experience sleep disturbances report more severe symptoms (Cong and Bian, 2022). A lack of rest can make your gut more sensitive to pain, increase inflammation, and even alter the helpful microbes in your digestive tract. Sleep can be disturbed for a number of reasons. Let's explore some of them and how they relate to gastrointestinal health.

Sleep Apnea

Sleep apnea is a condition where breathing repeatedly stops and starts during sleep. This can be caused by blocked airways from muscles that relax in the head and neck when sleeping, leading to low oxygen levels and resulting in numerous health consequences, including IBS symptom exacerbation. Low oxygen levels can disrupt the balance in the microbiome, while waking numerous times in the middle of the night can activate the stress response and increase inflammation in the body.

Insomnia

Insomnia is when you have difficulty falling and/or staying asleep. People who experience insomnia often report feeling fatigued and stressed. As with sleep apnea, poor sleep can lead to heightened visceral hypersensitivity and increased circulation of stress hormones. Insomnia can also reduce your resilience to stress and lead to difficulty coping with symptoms and following treatment plans.

Shift Work

Shift work refers to a work schedule where employees work outside of the standard 9-to-5 workday. Shifts often include evenings, overnights, or rotating shifts where work happens in the daytime on one shift and overnight on another shift. Shift work disrupts the body's circadian rhythm by altering normal sleep–wake cycles. This confuses the gut's internal clock, affecting digestion, gut motility, and microbial activity. Fatigue is a big component of shift work. These folks also tend to eat their meals at different times during the day than the average day worker, which can trigger IBS symptoms.

Jet Lag

Have you ever traveled to another time zone and couldn't keep your eyes open, even though the local time was right in the middle of the day? That fatigue is jet lag and it disrupts the body's internal clock, leading to a temporary change in sleep and wake times. Even though it is temporary, there might still be alterations to your microbiome.

When traveling, your eating patterns, food choices, and hydration status may change, and consequences might include bloating, excess gas, abdominal pain, and constipation.

In addition to sleep apnea, insomnia, shift work, and jet lag, anxiety and depression, IBS symptoms, and certain medications can disrupt sleep. While anxiety and depression fall into the "stress" trigger category, challenges from managing these diagnoses can lead to difficulty sleeping. Medications like steroids, cold remedies, and migraine reducers can alter sleep cycles. Though not typically common in IBS, if you experience overnight pain, bloating, nighttime accidents, or urgent trips to the bathroom, they can directly disrupt sleep. If you do experience overnight IBS symptoms, reach out to your doctor as these can be signs of other GI issues beyond IBS.

Living with IBS often feels like a puzzle where food is the most obvious piece, but it's not the only one. As we've explored, stress and sleep are significant factors that can contribute to the onset, frequency, and severity of symptoms. Understanding how these three triggers impact your IBS journey is key to gaining control over your symptoms and improving your quality of life.

Recognizing that IBS is not just about food can be empowering. It shifts the focus from restrictive diets to a more comprehensive and integrated approach to symptom management. Whether it's identifying specific food triggers, incorporating stress-reduction techniques, or prioritizing restorative sleep, each step you take brings you closer to relief and resilience.

In the next few chapters you will find tools to help you determine your triggers and manage your symptoms, whether they stem from food, stress, or poor sleep. You do not need to take this journey toward IBS management alone though—there are health professionals who have expertise in helping folks determine their symptom triggers and create a roadmap toward wellness.

6

Dietary Interventions to Manage Food-Related Triggers

In the last chapter we reviewed the three main triggers for IBS symptoms. While food gets blamed for digestive distress, not all food is to blame. In order to avoid eliminating possible suspects from your diet without reintroducing them when they are innocent bystanders, it's important to understand what types of foods will most likely lead to symptoms, if food is the cause. When looking at the research behind dietary interventions for managing irritable bowel syndrome, one diet stands out above all else with regard to alleviating the most common GI issues: the low-FODMAP diet.

A side note before delving into what a FODMAP is: I will use the term "diet" interchangeably with "dietary intervention" throughout this chapter. In our society, the word *diet* is typically seen as a weight-loss tool and weight loss is considered a means to health. In the weight-inclusive approach to care that I take, weight loss is not synonymous with health, nor a goal for symptom management. In fact, restrictive eating and intentional weight-loss activities can be the impetus for IBS. *Diet* was initially meant to define your pattern of eating. You may have heard of eating a *well-rounded diet* or a *balanced diet*, neither of which means restricting intake to make your body smaller. Diet culture co-opted these terms and they are now seen by most as phrases synonymous with restrictive eating. The purpose of a diet or dietary intervention as I see it (and as I hope you will come to embrace) is as a tool toward symptom management and an opportunity to take charge of what is within your control to care for your body with a chronic disease.

What the Heck is a FODMAP?

FODMAP stands for

Fermentable
Oligosaccharides
Disaccharides
Monosaccharides
And
Polyols

These are the chemical names for fermentable carbohydrates—the fibers, sugars, and starches that are indigestible or poorly absorbed in the GI tract. In people with IBS, eating them can lead to GI symptoms. The tricky thing is that not all people with IBS will be sensitive to FODMAPs, and those who are will not be sensitive to all of them. In fact, many people who experience symptoms after consuming high-FODMAP foods will be sensitive to only one or two of them. And it gets trickier: You can't tell by looking at a food whether it contains FODMAPs or high-FODMAP ingredients, and manufacturers rarely indicate if their product is low-FODMAP on the packaging. Trickier still is that even if you think you might be sensitive to high-FODMAP foods, you may not be an appropriate candidate for the diet.

Let's break down the low-FODMAP dietary intervention into digestible bits (pun intended!) so that if food is a trigger for you, you will understand the tool that will help you to best manage your symptoms. We'll begin with a deep dive into each FODMAP category, the different options for following the dietary intervention, how to implement it, and lastly, how to know if the low-FODMAP diet is the right tool for you.

Fermentable

Fermentable isn't one of the categories in the low-FODMAP diet but a term describing how certain carbohydrates are broken down during digestion. All carbohydrates are broken down by digestive enzymes in our saliva and stomach. For some carbohydrates, that's all that happens to them, and your body uses them for fuel.

In the case of fermentable carbohydrates, aka FODMAPs, these carbohydrates are then further broken down by microbes which use them for their fuel. The process of fermentation produces gas, which can lead to bloating, abdominal pain, and changes in bowel habits for people with IBS. Knowing which carbohydrates are fermentable is not intuitive—there has been much research and testing of many carbohydrate-containing foods to identify them and categorize them into carbohydrate types: oligosaccharides, disaccharides, monosaccharides, and polyols.

Oligosaccharides

Oligosaccharides are short chains of sugar molecules that our bodies cannot break down because we lack the enzymes to digest them. Instead, these carbohydrates pass into the large intestine, where gut bacteria ferment them, producing gas and other byproducts. There are two main types of oligosaccharides: fructans and galacto-oligosaccharides (GOS).

Examples of fructans	*Examples of GOS*
Wheat	Beans
Rye	Lentils
Barley	Peas
Onions	
Garlic	
An ingredient called inulin*	

* Inulin is a sweet, non-caloric, high-FODMAP, prebiotic fiber that is added to everything from fiber supplements to granola bars and yogurt.

Disaccharides

Disaccharides are made of two sugar molecules bonded together. The most common disaccharide that causes issues is lactose, the sugar found in milk. People who are lactose intolerant lack enough of the enzyme lactase, which is needed to break down lactose. A lactase deficiency can lead to lots of excess gas and changes in gut motility.

Examples of disaccharides
Milk from cows, sheep, and goats
Soft cheeses that have not been aged, like ricotta or cream cheese
Cottage cheese
Yogurt
Ice cream

Monosaccharides

Monosaccharides are single sugar molecules. Of them, the only one that is high-FODMAP is fructose, but only when it is above a 1:1 ratio with glucose. We refer to the high-FODMAP version of it as "excess fructose" because glucose helps fructose to be absorbed into the bloodstream. When there is not enough glucose, the remaining fructose molecules end up undigested in the large intestine and lead to symptoms of bloating, gas, and changes in bowel habits.

Examples of monosaccharides
Apples
Pears
Honey
Apricots
High-fructose corn syrup

Polyols

Polyols are sugar alcohols that are either naturally present in certain fruits and vegetables or added as artificial sweeteners. The most common high-FODMAP polyols are sorbitol and mannitol. Others end in -ol, like xylitol and maltitol. They are poorly absorbed in the gut and can draw water into the intestines, leading to diarrhea, or be fermented by gut bacteria, causing gas and bloating. Sugar alcohols are often included in medications but not at a level high enough to trigger symptoms in most cases, so there is no need to eliminate those medications when following the low-FODMAP diet.

Examples containing sorbitol	*Examples containing mannitol*
Peaches	Cauliflower
Watermelon	Mushrooms
Blackberries	Snow peas
Sugar-free gum and mints	

Although it is possible to have issues with multiple categories of FODMAPs, people with IBS who have food intolerances tend to have issues with only one category. For instance, say you feel symptoms develop from eating onions. If you have a second food trigger, it's more likely to be another fructan like garlic rather than a food with excess fructose like honey. In addition, there are some foods that have more than one FODMAP. Watermelon is high in fructans, excess fructose, and mannitol. Sounds convoluted and confusing, but there are tools that can help you with the low-FODMAP diet to make it less so. Before we get to the diet itself, let's look at why it is called the *low*-FODMAP diet and not the *no*-FODMAP diet.

Low-FODMAP, Not No-FODMAP

The low-FODMAP diet is portion-specific, meaning that some foods are low in FODMAPs until you get to a certain portion of that food, and once there, the concentration of FODMAPs is high enough to trigger symptoms if you are intolerant to that food. In the example above with watermelon, three teaspoons of watermelon per meal is considered low-FODMAP. Watermelon has elevated levels of fructans, excess fructose, and mannitol at one cup. Milk is low in lactose at three teaspoons, moderate in lactose at a quarter cup, and high in lactose and therefore high-FODMAP at one cup.

If I listed all of the foods available to us and their FODMAP content, this would be a much bigger book! Instead, the researchers at Monash University in Australia, the creators of the dietary intervention and the testing procedure for FODMAPs in food, have developed an app that contains all of the foods around the world that have been tested. Because our food comes from different climates, soils, and a host of other variables, they continue to test and retest food and update the portion sizes.

Every time a food is found to be high in FODMAPs or the amount of FODMAPs in the food is lower than initially thought, the researchers at Monash add it to the app. There are plenty of practitioners who have created handouts, books, and websites about the low-FODMAP diet and include a list of foods to avoid. The problem with these resources is that when Monash updates a food, adds a new high-FODMAP food, or finds that a food is lower in FODMAPs than previously thought, the resources from the practitioner become out of date. Many of these resources are accessed by people with IBS looking to follow the low-FODMAP diet. Because this is a relatively new dietary intervention (created in 2005) and changes to the food list come fairly frequently, the resources found online almost always contain outdated information that can lead to unnecessary restriction or the inclusion of a possible trigger food once considered low-FODMAP but now found to be high. The gold standard for determining whether a food is low- or high-FODMAP is the Monash University FODMAP Diet app.

The Low-FODMAP Diet

The low-FODMAP dietary intervention is a three-phase program. These phases are meant to help you to reduce your intake of FODMAP-containing foods temporarily to allow symptoms and inflammation to subside and give your gut–brain axis time to rest and reset, reintroduce the high-FODMAP foods to see which, if any, are your triggers (remember that food is only one trigger—stress and poor sleep are the other two musketeers), and then create a personalized plan of foods that will keep your symptoms at bay while liberalizing your diet as much as possible. Since its inception, there have been some alternative methods to implementing the diet. We will look at some of them, but let's start with the basics by going through the three phases: the elimination phase, the reintroduction phase, and the personalization phase.

Phase One: The Elimination Phase

In this first phase, the goal is to reduce the amount of FODMAPs you are consuming. This is done by eliminating all high-FODMAP foods from your diet. This phase is the shortest phase of the intervention as you should eliminate these foods for only two to six weeks. During this time, keep a log that includes the foods you chose to eat, whether you experienced symptoms, what your bowel habits were like, as well as any additional information about your stress levels and sleep quality. Collecting this information gives you the opportunity to see if there are positive, negative, or neutral outcomes over time.

At the two-week mark, you should be able to tell if the diet has made a remarkable difference, a little bit of a difference, or no difference at all. If you experience positive changes such as a reduction in bloating and gas, firmer bowel movements (for those with diarrhea), or less straining when moving your bowels (for those with constipation), then it is clear that the low-FODMAP diet is working, and it is time to move to the reintroduction phase. If you look through your log and notice no difference in symptoms, then the diet is not working for you, food is most likely not your IBS trigger, and you can abandon the diet and go back to the way you were eating before the elimination phase. For some, the results are unclear. Maybe you see a slight difference in symptoms but not enough to tell whether it's working or not. In this case, you can stay on the elimination phase for up to six weeks.

One issue I see with clients is that when they are on the elimination diet and it is working well, they are loath to move to reintroduction. They finally feel relief and don't want to add back any food that might bring back discomfort. I totally understand that, but there are two reasons for reintroduction. The first is that the elimination phase can be restrictive and can limit your ability to eat socially when avoiding foods like wheat, milk, onions, and garlic, to name a few. The second has to do with your microbiome. Foods high in FODMAPs are also high in prebiotic fiber, which is the fan-favorite source of nutrients for our microbes. By removing practically all sources of prebiotic fiber from your diet, you can throw your whole microbiome off balance, and over time this can lead to a whole host of GI symptoms—exactly what the low-FODMAP diet aims to avoid. In order to avoid the risk of food aversion and get you back to eating all foods (with the exception of what is truly triggering your IBS symptoms), move to the reintroduction phase after 2–6 weeks (Halmos and Gibson, 2019).

Research shows that 50–80 percent of people who follow the low-FODMAP diet experience improvement in their IBS symptoms (Nanayakkara et al., 2016). That's wonderful news for so many! Unfortunately, there are still that 20–50 percent that don't see improvement. If you are one of them, do not fret. This means that you have ruled out one of the three main triggers for IBS symptoms. It's now time to focus on managing stress and/or improving sleep. There are also non-diet interventions that can help with symptom management that we will explore in the next chapter. If you happen to be one of the 50–80 percent that do find symptom improvement while on the elimination phase, then food is definitely a trigger for you. It is now time to move on to the reintroduction phase and determine which one or ones are the culprit.

Phase Two: The Reintroduction Phase

The reintroduction phase is commonly overlooked. You might see a healthcare practitioner who suggests you try the low-FODMAP diet. They give you a handout or a link to a webpage with some information about foods to avoid and tell you to follow it and see if it helps. In many of these cases, there is no follow-up after the initial suggestion about the diet and you are left to believe that if it works, you stay on it for the foreseeable future, and if it doesn't work, you'll just have to deal with your symptoms.

The low-FODMAP diet was created with three phases for a reason: determine if food is the issue, figure out which foods are causing the issue, and liberalize the diet as much as possible once that information is available. The reintroduction phase is the most important step in the diet because it's where we find out which food or foods were causing symptoms. While the reintroduction phase has not been studied as deeply as the elimination phase, there are some studies and best practices by skilled practitioners on the most effective way to implement it (Chey et al., 2022). It is a systematic reintroduction of food so that we can determine what food and how much of that food causes GI distress.

There are a few ways to begin the reintroduction phase. One is to reintroduce food by FODMAP category, for instance starting with testing fructans before moving on to polyols. Another way is to choose foods on an individual basis by selecting a food that you don't think will cause symptoms or a food that will make eating easier for you. For instance, you might not think you have any trouble digesting wheat and would like to start with that food because you would like to have a successful reintroduction on your first attempt. Or you might start with garlic because it would make eating out easier for you and you tend to eat meals away from home quite frequently. Whichever path you choose is up to you. Eventually, you will be reintroducing those foods, so the order does not matter.

To begin, choose a food and then reintroduce it to your low-FODMAP diet one time per day for three days in a row. Over the course of the three days, the portion size will increase from a small portion that is enough to make the food high in FODMAPs, then to a medium portion the following day, and then a full portion on the third day. A full portion is not a specific measurement, it is the amount of the food you would normally eat in a meal. Say you choose to reintroduce wheat and select sandwich bread to do so. When you eat a sandwich, you normally make it with two slices of bread, so let's work backwards from your full portion.

Day 3: Two slices of bread
Day 2: One slice of bread
Day 1: ½ a slice of bread

But what if you love and only eat club sandwiches? Those contain three slices of bread. All you would need to do is set your third day at three slices and work backwards: two slices on Day 2 and one slice on Day 1. If you choose to start with apples and you typically eat a whole apple, then Day 1 would be one-third of an apple, Day 2 would be two-thirds of an apple, and Day 3 would be the whole apple.

Once you've chosen your first food to try and determined your portion size for each day, you can get started. Incorporate that food into one of your meals or snacks one time in the day. It's a good idea to continue that food and symptom log you began during the elimination phase to keep track of any changes in your symptoms or bowel habits. Each day note whether you've had any of your symptoms return to the level that would make eating this reintroduced food uncomfortable for your GI system.

If at any time during the three days you have symptoms that match this description, stop your reintroduction. For instance, if you have the food on Day 1 and you are fine but on Day 2 you experience abdominal cramping and bloating, you do not need to move on to Day 3 and we would consider this an unsuccessful reintroduction. If you eat the food on Days 1 and 2 without issue but have symptoms on Day 3, you have some new information: your Day 2 portion is what you are able to tolerate per meal. That doesn't mean that you can only consume it once per day. For instance, if you reintroduce one slice of bread on Day 2 and two slices on Day 3 and have symptoms, then you will be able to tolerate one slice of bread every three to four hours each day. You do not need to avoid it completely. However, if you eat the food on all three days without any major GI distress, then we would consider this a successful reintroduction.

When you have encountered an unsuccessful reintroduction, put it on a list and avoid eating it, but only for a short time. As your gut continues to heal from inflammation and your most recent flare, it is possible to reintroduce a food from your list of unsuccessful reintroductions. It is suggested to wait three months and try again. In my experience with the low-FODMAP diet, I had a number of unsuccessful reintroductions at first, but now I have only two high-FODMAP foods that still trigger symptoms years later. The good news is, I can eat them with the help of some non-dietary interventions that I will share in the next chapter.

If you have a successful reintroduction, go ahead and jump for joy! Adding back a food that was once thought to be causing symptoms but which you now know without a doubt is safe for you to eat with no GI distress is cause for celebration. Unfortunately, that celebration will be short-lived as that food will be added to

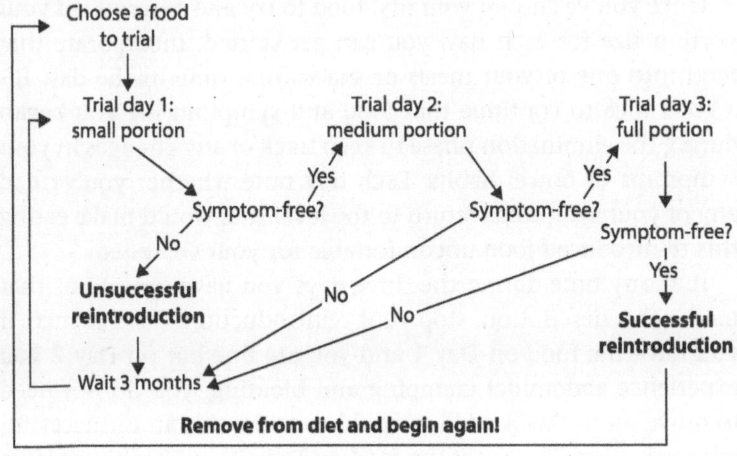

Figure 6.1 The reintroduction phase

your list of successful reintroductions but removed from your diet as you continue the reintroduction process.

After reintroducing a food, whether it was a success or not, it needs to leave your system before you try the next food. At the end of the three-day food trial, you begin another three-day period called the washout period. These are days where the trialed food is removed from your diet and you go back to eating only low-FODMAP foods. This is especially necessary for those with constipation-predominant IBS to give the body time to clear out the first food before starting the second. At the end of the washout period, the reintroduction of the next food begins.

It is not necessary to reintroduce every food that is high-FODMAP, especially if there are some that you don't eat, don't like, or don't have access to. It is important, however, to reintroduce all of the foods that you like, ate regularly, and want to be able to eat without worry in the future. If you think about how long that list is, it will take a very long time to complete the reintroduction phase. The good news is that reintroducing a couple of foods from each FODMAP category will provide you with enough information to make assumptions about whether you can tolerate other foods within that category.

For instance, if you were to reintroduce foods from the excess fructose category—the monosaccharides—and trialed mangoes and honey and had a successful reintroduction of both foods, it would be safe to assume that you would be able to tolerate high-fructose corn syrup in soda or candy. The only exception is within the oligosaccharide category. Fructans and galacto-oligosaccharides have such varied concentrations of FODMAPs that you cannot glean information from one food and apply it to the rest. Therefore, you should reintroduce wheat, garlic, onion, and beans, if you consume these foods, one at a time.

If you trial two foods from a FODMAP group and you are able to tolerate one but not the other, that might be due to portion size or FODMAP concentration within the food. When this happens, trial a third food from the group or look back in your log to see if the unsuccessful food was trialed when you were experiencing a non-food IBS trigger like stress or poor sleep.

During reintroduction, the trialed food can be eaten raw or cooked as FODMAP content doesn't tend to change. For instance, if you were to test garlic, you could add it raw to a salad dressing or sauté it with your favorite low-FODMAP vegetable. You could also trial canned or tinned peaches instead of fresh peaches if they are not in season.

For foods with more than one FODMAP in them, leave them off your initial reintroduction phase. Apples, for instance, are high in both excess fructose and sorbitol, and mushrooms are high in fructans and mannitol. If you trial a food like that and you have an unsuccessful reintroduction, you will not be able to use that information to make assumptions about other foods high in those FODMAP categories because you won't know which FODMAP caused your symptoms to reappear or if it was both that triggered you. Best practice suggests that you first trial foods with a single FODMAP from each category before moving on to foods with multiple FODMAPs. There are cases, however, where you might want to trial an apple because it is your favorite food before trialing foods from the excess fructose and sorbitol groups like honey and cherries, respectively.

Ideally, reintroduction should take place when you are calm, happy, and well rested. Because it is possible to have triggers beyond food like stress and poor sleep, you may find that your symptoms return before you've started a trial. In these cases, it is best to reintroduce foods when you are not experiencing symptoms because it will be difficult to discern whether the symptoms are due to the reintroduction of a high-FODMAP food or because you had a hard time sleeping the night before.

This phase can be done all at once or you can take breaks. Taking breaks looks like this: You reintroduced wheat, garlic, and milk and added them to your successful reintroduction list. Before trialing the next food on your list, you would like to go out for Italian food, so you take a break from reintroduction and order pasta with oil and garlic and have ricotta cheesecake for dessert. The food is so delicious and the portions so large that you have leftovers and plan to eat them over the weekend. Once you are done with your leftovers, you feel ready to go back to reintroduction, so you do a three-day washout by removing wheat, garlic, and milk from your diet and go back to the low-FODMAP diet. After the three days, you trial the next food on your list.

Taking a break gives you the opportunity to eat the foods that you have successfully reintroduced, but it also slows the process of reintroduction. It is your journey toward IBS management and you get to choose how you will move through the phases. The most important step, though, is beginning the reintroduction phase and adding food back into your diet for the sake of your microbiome and quality of life.

Gluten or Fructan Intolerance?

Many people believe that the low-FODMAP diet is a gluten-free diet, but they would be wrong. Gluten is a protein found in wheat, rye, and barley. It's what gives structure to baked goods and chewiness to bread and pizza crust. While gluten is in the three grains that are avoided during the elimination phase, it is not their gluten content but their fructan content that is the reason for restriction. Remember that the F in FODMAP stands for fermentable and that the O, D, M and P stand for carbohydrates. Fructans fall into the oligosaccharide category.

The low-FODMAP diet is not gluten-free. There are foods that contain wheat like soy sauce, seitan, and sourdough bread that are low in FODMAPs and allowed during the elimination phase. If you are sensitive to wheat, rye, or barley, and you and your provider have ruled out celiac disease, you can proceed with determining if it is the protein or the carbohydrate in these grains that fuels your symptoms.

During the elimination phase, you can eat a gluten-free diet, substituting the gluten-containing products for gluten-free alternatives. When you begin the reintroduction phase, trial sourdough bread before testing back any other gluten-containing product. During the process of making sourdough, the microbes in the starter dough use the fructans to create that tangy taste. The end result is a low-fructan but gluten-containing wheat product. If, during the reintroduction to sourdough, you are symptom-free, then you are most likely able to tolerate gluten in wheat products. You may want to test wheat bread or pasta separately to confirm your tolerance. If you have an unsuccessful reintroduction experience with sourdough bread, it will indicate that you have a gluten sensitivity. This may be temporary, so consider retrialing a gluten-containing product in three months.

Phase Three: The Personalization Phase

The personalization phase is the final phase and the one that you will live within as long as you have food triggers. The elimination phase reduced fermentable carbohydrates that might have been contributing to your symptoms. The reintroduction phase guided you through pinpointing which foods were to blame. The personalization phase is a combination of both the elimination and reintroduction phases in that your diet during this phase is the low-FODMAP diet plus the foods you were able to successfully reintroduce. For some, this may look like their eating pattern before beginning the dietary intervention with only one or two foods removed. For others, it may look like the low-FODMAP diet with only a handful of foods added back. You will not have to avoid your unsuccessfully trialed foods for the rest of your life.

In fact, the longer you are in the personalization phase, the more likely you are to be able to reintroduce foods that were initially unsuccessful.

While in the personalization phase, it is a good idea to go back to the reintroduction phase about every three months and retrial the foods that triggered symptoms during their first reintroduction. Being in the personalization phase continues to give your gut time to heal from inflammation and irritation due to symptoms caused by high-FODMAP trigger foods. You may not be able to tolerate a whole apple on your first try, but maybe in three months you will be able to tolerate half an apple per meal and in six months it may be the whole apple!

When I went through the low-FODMAP diet, I had so many failed reintroductions. My IBS was caused by my recurrent *C. diff* infection, which activated significant inflammation in my gut. My first eating pattern in my personalization phase was limited compared to where I am today, but it was so much more expansive than it had been when I was removing foods without knowing for sure that they were the culprits. Fast-forward to today, after a number of reintroductions from my unsuccessful list, and I can comfortably eat garlic, cauliflower, apples, and cherries without issue. It took a few tries with apples and cherries, but I am happy to report that I now look forward to cherry season each spring. There are still some foods on my unsuccessful list that continue to be triggers for me, but knowing the cause of my symptoms and that they will be temporary, I am willing to continue to reintroduce them.

I hope that in your journey toward discovering your food triggers you will be empowered to continue liberalizing your diet as your IBS symptoms decrease. Once you have been through the low-FODMAP diet, you know which foods will and will not trigger symptoms. If you do experience symptoms and you have not ingested those foods, do not blame food. Instead, look to see if something else might be leading to symptoms.

Now that you are well acquainted with the low-FODMAP diet, let's look at the alternate forms of the diet.

FODMAP Gentle

After about a decade of research and use of the low-FODMAP diet, the creators discovered a trend. Among those who completed the reintroduction phase, there were high-FODMAP foods that proved to be the most common triggers. The researchers studied whether removing just these most common food triggers, rather than all high-FODMAP foods, would be as effective as the original low-FODMAP diet, but with far less restriction and more ease of use. To their pleasant surprise, they found that people following the FODMAP Gentle version of the low-FODMAP diet had a high success rate in identifying their food triggers. This discovery has made the low-FODMAP diet more manageable for people with IBS to follow as the list of foods is quite short compared with the app filled with hundreds of foods. Here are the foods to avoid during the elimination phase of the FODMAP Gentle alternative intervention.

Food group	*Foods to avoid during elimination*
Dairy	Cow's milk and yogurt
Grains	Wheat and rye
Vegetables	Onions, leek bulb, garlic, cauliflower, and mushrooms
Fruits	Apples, pears, stone fruit (peaches, plums, nectarines, cherries, and mangoes), and dried fruit (e.g. dates, raisins, prunes)
Protein	Beans and peas

The FODMAP Gentle uses the same three phases as the original diet. It is important to use a food and symptom log with this version as well to look for improvements in symptoms, but also to see if there are times when symptoms arise. If you notice that you are improving but do have symptoms on occasion, it is possible that you are sensitive to a high-FODMAP food that is not part of the FODMAP Gentle intervention. Your dietitian or trained healthcare practitioner can review your log and see what that high-FODMAP food might be and add it to your list of foods to avoid during elimination to determine whether it is a trigger. The reintroduction phase is followed as it is in the original and any additional foods added to your elimination phase will go through a trial to determine their impact on your GI system.

The FODMAP Gentle diet can be further liberalized in a couple of categories. It recommends avoiding cow's milk and yogurt during the elimination phase because of the disaccharide lactose, but there are versions of cow's milk and yogurt on the market that are lactose-free, and you can have those products during reintroduction. The other category that has some wiggle room is the grains group. Although you are avoiding wheat, you can include real sourdough bread. Real sourdough bread is made from a starter that contains microbes that consume the fructans and give sourdough that tangy flavor. The microbes essentially feed off the high-FODMAP ingredient, making sourdough bread a low-FODMAP food. Real sourdough bread does not contain yeast or vinegar—these ingredients do not break down the fructans and sourdough loaves that contain them are still high in FODMAPs. Reading labels is important when choosing sourdough bread in a grocery store so that you know what kind of sourdough you are consuming.

Cherry Picking

Sometimes, the low-FODMAP diet is not an appropriate tool for someone with IBS. For instance, if you are already following a restrictive dietary intervention to manage another diagnosis, like diabetes, adding to that restriction can make eating at home and socially quite difficult. An alternative to the low-FODMAP diet and the FODMAP Gentle variation is "cherry picking." This term was coined by Patsy Catsos, a registered dietitian who was one of the first to use the low-FODMAP diet in the U.S. Cherry picking works by having a registered dietitian or FODMAP-trained healthcare professional look through your food and symptom log and find possible culprits for your GI distress and suggest eliminating only one or two FODMAPs at a time while offering nutritionally equivalent substitutions, especially if you are already restricted in a particular food group due to following another eating pattern for disease management.

You can also cherry pick in addition to the FODMAP Gentle diet. As mentioned earlier, if you are still having symptoms after consuming certain meals, a registered dietitian can use your food and symptom log to identify other high-FODMAP foods that might be contributing to symptoms and add those to the elimination phase of FODMAP Gentle.

I have done this with my own clients. When avocado was all the rage, people were eating lots of them, particularly at breakfast. Avocado on toast with an egg was a popular dish and one to two avocados could be consumed at a meal. Avocados contain polyols—specifically sorbitol—and are at a high-FODMAP level at 4.5 tablespoons, or about half of an average avocado. Having one to two avocados in a meal provides a high concentration of FODMAPs at one sitting. Cherry picking in this case might mean removing avocado, but it also might mean reducing the intake of avocado per meal to its low-FODMAP portion size, three tablespoons. That small change can make all the difference in your symptoms.

Appropriate Candidates for the Low-FODMAP Diet

It may seem like anyone with IBS would be an appropriate candidate for the low-FODMAP diet, but there are more circumstances where the low-FODMAP diet would not be the best tool for symptom management. In order to determine if you would be a good candidate for the low-FODMAP diet, consider the following criteria before beginning.

Have a Diagnosis

This may seem obvious to you now, but it is imperative to get a proper diagnosis in order to rule out other diseases and disorders that may have similar symptoms. Using the low-FODMAP diet without first addressing any alarm features may lead to a delay in treating something that may get progressively worse if not properly dealt with. The low-FODMAP diet may work without a diagnosis if you do indeed have IBS, but that doesn't mean that you don't also have other issues going on. Seek confirmation of diagnoses before beginning any dietary intervention.

Be Well Nourished

The low-FODMAP diet eliminates fermentable carbohydrates found in some grains, fruits, vegetables, dairy products, nuts, and beans. Beyond fermentable carbohydrates, these foods provide a whole host of vitamins, minerals, antioxidants, and fiber which support your health. Eating a well-rounded diet allows for access to all nutrients, but the low-FODMAP elimination phase can be quite restrictive and limit access to some of them. Beginning the diet in a nourished state will protect your health during this temporary period of restriction. One way to tell if you are well nourished is through your blood work and your symptoms. For instance, a zinc deficiency can lead to diarrhea while a magnesium deficiency might contribute to constipation. In addition to blood work, eating patterns and your relationship with food and eating can be a key to nourishment. People with disordered eating behaviors or eating disorder diagnoses struggle with being well nourished. Being well nourished may improve GI symptoms, so correcting any nutrient deficiencies prior to beginning the low-FODMAP diet can be quite helpful in symptom management.

Inappropriate Candidates for the Low-FODMAP Diet

There are far more criteria for finding that someone is an inappropriate candidate for the low-FODMAP diet than there are for it being a good fit. This is why it's great that we now have access to the FODMAP Gentle and cherry-picking options. We've discussed having a diagnosis and being well nourished as criteria for appropriate candidates, so the opposite would be criteria for inappropriate candidates—those without a diagnosis and/or those who have nutrient deficiencies. Some of the other criteria that rule out the use of the low-FODMAP diet include candidates who fall into the following groups.

Children

Restrictive diets of any kind can trigger maladaptive eating patterns in children. We want to *always* be very careful of the limitations we put on children with regard to diet. If a child has been diagnosed with IBS, it is best to cherry pick and substitute, and to use non-diet interventions with the help of a registered dietitian.

The Elderly

In many cases, the elderly lack access to technology to use the most updated food lists that are available only in the Monash Low-FODMAP app. In addition, there could be some financial strain from being on a fixed income, and buying food that they will consume for only a short time may not be feasible. This population is at a higher risk of malnourishment, so prolonged restriction of any type is not recommended for our seniors.

Those Currently on a Diet

If you are already following a dietary intervention for another diagnosis, or if you are participating in intentional weight-loss activities, you shouldn't try the low-FODMAP diet as it would introduce more restriction and put you at a higher risk of malnutrition. There are certain dietary interventions where the low-FODMAP diet can work in tandem (for example, the Mediterranean diet for heart health), but there are far more where adding in more restriction, especially in terms of fad diets (for instance, keto, paleo, intermittent fasting), would cause more harm than good. Removing any unnecessary restriction prior to beginning the low-FODMAP diet could make you an appropriate candidate. Check with your healthcare professional who prescribed a dietary intervention for other diagnoses to see if the two interventions can be used in tandem to support both health issues.

Disordered Eating and Eating Disorders

Before beginning any dietary intervention, you should be screened for disordered eating patterns and eating disorders. Among those with diagnosed eating disorders, up to 98 percent have functional GI issues, so it is common in my practice to find people with poor relationships with food and their bodies who also have IBS. Restrictive eating in any form can disrupt the microbiome, slowing your gut motility and altering hunger and fullness signals, which can then lead to a continuation of maladaptive eating patterns.

Intentional weight-loss activities like following a restrictive diet that eliminates food groups or reduces portion sizes mimicking starvation have been touted as "healthy" behaviors but are in fact *disordered* behaviors that have been normalized by a society convinced that thinness equals health. Dieting is one of the most common triggers for eating disorders, resulting in a slippery slope of behaviors, beliefs and attitudes about food and body that increase the risk of cardiovascular issues, GI distress, nutrient deficiencies, and death. Eating disorders are no joke. If your GI practitioner is not screening you before offering the low-FODMAP diet, they are doing you a dangerous disservice. If you think you might have disordered eating tendencies, seek support and a diagnosis from a mental health professional.

If you're unsure whether you fall into this category, try this self-assessment and speak to your healthcare provider about next steps and alternate interventions.

	Yes	*No*
Do you ever reduce your food or calorie intake to lose weight?		
Do you avoid certain foods or food groups because eating them will lead to weight gain?		
Do you ever feel guilty after eating?		
Do you ever hide food or eat in secret?		
Have you ever compensated for eating by vomiting, using laxatives, or exercising?		
Do you ever fast for eight consecutive hours or more while you are awake other than for religious observances?		
Do thoughts about food or calories often distract you from what you are doing?		
Do you ever choose clothing that hides parts of your body you deem "not good enough"?		
Do you often have negative thoughts about the size and shape of your body?		

If you answered "yes" to even one of these questions, you may have disordered eating tendencies. If you answered "yes" to more than one, it may be worth reaching out to an eating disorder-informed mental health practitioner to be evaluated. Reducing intake, food group restriction, fasting, and exercising to "burn" what you've eaten have unfortunately become part of mainstream diet culture, but don't be fooled: eating disorders are serious medical conditions that can lead to a decline in cardiovascular, gastrointestinal, and bone health, and, sadly, death. If you suspect you have a disordered relationship with food, please seek help.

Those Not Interested

When I am assessing a client for the appropriateness of the low-FODMAP diet, I ask them how willing they will be to eliminate certain foods, knowing that it will change how they prepare or acquire meals. Even though the intervention has a high rate of success, some people are just not interested in changing their diet for the sake of symptom management. And that's okay. If the thought of having to remove foods like bread and garlic from your diet seems impossible, and you know you will not stick to an elimination period, then the low-FODMAP diet is not for you. Rest assured, there are other tools that can manage food-related triggers without a dietary intervention for those who are inappropriate candidates for whatever reason.

Keeping a Log

Whether you choose the low-FODMAP diet in its original form, the FODMAP Gentle, or cherry picking, keeping a log throughout each phase will provide you with data for determining what your food triggers are, how they impact your bowel habits and other symptoms, and whether or not they are improving throughout the phases. You can keep your log in a spreadsheet or on your phone, but it can be as simple as keeping it with a good old-fashioned pen and notepad.

Start with the date and the phase of the intervention that you are in. Include what time you ate and what foods, condiments, and beverages you ingested during that eating opportunity. You do not need to measure or note portions of your foods in your log. Weighing and measuring food can evolve into a disordered eating behavior and are unnecessary for this dietary intervention. Next, include any symptoms you experience. This may not line up with meal and snack times, so note the time when you notice the symptoms. Some high-FODMAP foods can take a long time to ferment. It's more likely that your symptoms will occur within hours rather than seconds or minutes of your meal or snack.

You will also want to keep track of your bowel habits. Include information about how often you moved them, or if you are constipated, if you needed to strain to move them, or didn't move them at all. Note the appearance and consistency of your stool and if there are any alarming features like blood or mucus.

Lastly, you might want to include whether you had a good night's sleep and if you were having a stressful day. Remember that food isn't the only trigger for IBS symptoms. For those who don't see a benefit from following the low-FODMAP diet, tracking sleep and stress may be the key to what is causing symptoms to flare.

Throughout each phase, your log can be a helpful tool for collecting information about how food impacts your body. When I am working with clients, I let them know that I do not need to see their logs. Instead, I ask them about what insights they have gained from keeping the log. Sometimes, when we think someone will look at our food intake and bowel habits, we might not enter all of the information for fear of being judged or embarrassed. I always assure my clients that I am not the food police—more like a food cheerleader or a symptom sleuth—and all the information contained in their log tells a story. What you leave out might be the key to finding answers and it would be a shame to miss out on the opportunity to feel better and calm your flare.

The low-FODMAP diet is an excellent and effective tool for determining food triggers for IBS. It provides a personalized approach to finding the foods that are causing your symptoms, thus allowing you to ultimately liberalize your diet. Best of all, it is backed by science. In the almost two decades it has been around, there have been hundreds of research studies testing its efficacy.

While the benefits of the low-FODMAP diet are substantial, there are some drawbacks as well. It can be tricky to follow, especially with the ever growing and changing food list that is only available through Monash University's proprietary app. This may leave the technologically challenged folks without access to the intervention. If you are able to follow it, it can also be restrictive and limited in certain nutrients, putting some populations at risk.

If you are an appropriate candidate for the low-FODMAP diet and find answers, that's great news, and you now know what you need to do to minimize symptoms. But if you don't find food triggers, or if you do but eliminating them from your diet doesn't reduce all of your symptoms, a non-dietary intervention may be of help to you. In the next chapter, we will explore ways to manage symptoms beyond dietary interventions.

7

Non-Dietary Interventions for Symptom Management from Food, Stress, and Sleep

Irritable bowel syndrome is a chronic disease without a cure. There are tools that can help you manage symptoms in your quest to reduce the frequency, duration, and intensity of flares, but there is nothing you can do that will completely prevent flares. If food is the source of your triggers, *and* you are an appropriate candidate for the low-FODMAP diet, *and* you find relief from removing those foods from your diet, *and* you notice a reduction in the frequency, duration, and intensity of your flares, then you are among the lucky minority of people with IBS.

Most of us who do find that food is a trigger and are appropriate candidates for the low-FODMAP diet will still have symptoms that arise that are not connected to our trigger foods. Then, there are those of us who don't find relief from the low-FODMAP diet and manage flares from other triggers such as stress and poor sleep in other ways. If you fall into this segment of the IBS population, you'll need other interventions beyond the low-FODMAP diet for symptom management and improving your quality of life.

Although there is no cure for IBS, there are a number of tools with which you can fill your IBS toolbox. There are gut-directed psychotherapies for reconnecting the gut–brain communication and relieving symptoms that are stress-induced, prescriptions and over-the-counter medications and supplements to manage diarrhea, constipation, gas, and other motility disturbances, and behavior modifications to improve symptoms triggered by sleep as well as slow motility and pelvic floor dysfunction. In this chapter, we will explore the tools that are evidenced-based and that are backed by research so that you can begin to confidently experiment with tools that are safe and effective.

Managing Stress-Related Triggers

The gut and brain are intricately connected through the communication pathway known as the gut–brain axis. When stress or anxiety trigger your symptoms, it is because of the miscommunication that takes place along this pathway. There are a number of psychological modalities that can specifically support the healthy function of the gut–brain axis and reduce the triggers initiated by stress. These include gut-directed hypnotherapy (GHD), cognitive behavioral therapy (CBT), and mindfulness.

Gut-Directed Hypnotherapy

Gut-directed hypnotherapy is a form of therapy that uses hypnosis to help manage the symptoms of irritable bowel syndrome. This therapy is based on regulating the connection between the gut and the brain to improve the function of the digestive system. You might think of hypnosis as a parlor trick where people cluck like chickens or think that they aren't wearing any clothes, but there are medical uses for hypnotherapy as a powerful form of suggestion that, for example, helps people quit smoking. In IBS, gut-directed hypnotherapy focuses on improving gut function but also on reducing pain signals. GDH also works to quiet that drama queen, visceral hypersensitivity.

In GDH for IBS, a trained hypnotherapist guides you into a relaxed state and then uses suggestion and imagery to reduce symptoms. This type of therapy typically involves several sessions over a period of several weeks. Unfortunately, depending on where you live, you might have a difficult time finding practitioners trained in gut-directed hypnotherapy. There is, however, an app-based version of GDH that has been shown in research to significantly reduce IBS symptoms of pain, irregular bowel habits, and also anxiety. App-based GDH offers an affordable and accessible alternative to visiting a practitioner in an office with all of the same benefits. I have had clients remark that gut-directed hypnotherapy reduced their abdominal pain and frequent trips to the bathroom within a few weeks of beginning the program. For best results, find a quiet spot to relax while listening to 15 minutes of guided imagery and suggestion each day for the recommended length of the program.

Cognitive Behavioral Therapy

The theory of cognitive behavioral therapy focuses on changing the negative thoughts and behaviors that might be exacerbating symptoms. People who work in high-stress jobs, juggle lots of responsibilities in their daily lives, or fret about how their symptoms will interfere in their daily activities might benefit from reframing thoughts and changing behaviors. CBT supports this through a number of components. First is education about the relationship between stress and IBS symptoms and how to identify triggers. Once you understand what stressors can trigger IBS, you can learn and practice skills that can reduce those stressors, be they thoughts or behaviors. Cognitive restructuring teaches you how to identify negative thoughts and restructure them, while behavioral strategies offer tools to avoid or change situations that trigger stress. Calming techniques such as diaphragmatic breathing and progressive muscle relaxation help to reduce stress and anxiety.

Diaphragmatic breathing is an easy tool to master. It's as simple as slow, deep, belly breathing. If you have ever taken a yoga class, you've practiced diaphragmatic breathing. To start, take a slow, deep breath and let the air expand your belly outward. If your belly is not moving out and instead your shoulders are moving up, relax those shoulders and try again. Once you have that deep breath slowly inhaled, you can hold it for a few seconds and then exhale it just as slowly as you inhaled, and pause at the end before taking the next deep breath. Some diaphragmatic breathing includes counting the seconds of the inhalation of breath, the hold, and the exhale. It can be a count where the inhale is a shorter duration than the exhale, or where the inhale, hold, and exhale are equal. The latter is referred to as square breathing and can be quite relaxing. Try it by counting to four on the inhale, the hold, the exhale, and the pause. Repeat it a few times and note whether you feel calmer and more present.

Mindfulness

Mindfulness is the practice of paying attention to the present moment on purpose with curious observation. That means noticing what you're thinking, feeling, or sensing right now—whether it's your breath, the way your body feels, or the sounds around you—without judgment. Doing so helps you to acknowledge what you are feeling in the present moment without focusing on what will happen in the future. Practicing mindfulness can help calm your nervous system, which may lead to fewer or less intense IBS symptoms and flares.

There are many ways to practice mindfulness. One simple way is through mindful breathing. You can sit quietly, close your eyes if you feel comfortable, and slowly breathe in and out while noticing how your breath feels. This is different from diaphragmatic breathing in that you are not altering your breath, just observing it. Another technique is a body scan, where you focus your attention on different parts of your body, starting from your toes and moving up to your head. This helps you notice tension and release it.

Mindfulness can also be part of everyday activities. For example, you can go on a mindful walk by paying attention to how the ground feels under your feet, the movement of your body, and the sights and sounds around you. You can even shower mindfully by noticing the temperature of the water, the feeling of scrubbing your scalp, and steps you move through to cleanse your body. These mindfulness practices help you stay present and reduce stress by avoiding thoughts of what could have been or what might happen in the future. Letting your brain focus on the "what ifs" can lead to increased stress, and mindfulness helps to reduce the risk of this trigger.

We lead busy lives and not all stress management tools can be used wherever you are, but diaphragmatic breathing is something that you can do anywhere. I practice at traffic lights. Anytime I am sitting at a red light, I have time to take a few slow, deep breaths. Even if stress is not your trigger for IBS, you will be surprised by how good it feels to take a moment and just breathe.

Gut-based psychotherapies are backed by research suggesting that they can lead to significant improvements in symptoms and quality of life (Black et al., 2020; Peters, Gibson and Halmos, 2023). However, it's important to note that, just like with the low-FODMAP diet, not all people will benefit from these approaches.

But experimenting with them is the only way to know if they help, so give them a try.

Managing Poor Sleep

We discussed the main causes of poor sleep habits in Chapter 5, including sleep apnea, insomnia, shift work, and jet lag. Even a small change like staying up until midnight on New Year's Eve when you normally go to bed at 10 pm can be enough to impact your circadian rhythm and trigger IBS symptoms. If you think you have sleep apnea or have been diagnosed already, it's important to follow your treatment plan in order to get restful, effective sleep. You might need to wear a CPAP (continuous positive airway pressure) machine or a mouth guard to support your airways. Even though these items might seem like a bother to use, long-term, untreated sleep apnea can impact your IBS symptoms as well as your cardiovascular and brain health.

If you have insomnia, there are tools available to make sleeping easier, including prescription and over-the-counter medications and cognitive behavioral therapy specifically designed for insomnia. Practicing good sleep hygiene can also improve your sleep quality and, in turn, your IBS symptoms.

Developing a sleep hygiene regimen includes creating an atmosphere in your bedroom that is conducive to sleep. This might include lowering the temperature until the room is cool, closing the shades and turning off the overhead lights to provide darkness, and maybe most importantly, reducing brain stimulation close to bedtime, especially through the use of screens like a smartphone or computer.

If you work shifts and you have any control over your schedule, try to keep within the same shift times each week. If you sleep during the daytime, consider installing blackout shades or curtains in your bedroom or getting a high-quality sleep mask to mimic the nighttime. You may need to use earplugs or white noise to drown out sounds around your home during the day, such as children and pets, or doorbells and passing vehicles. It may also help to avoid caffeine during the last half of your shift so that you will be able to fall asleep without a stimulant in your system.

Those who are lucky enough to travel and get jet-lagged would benefit from gradually adjusting sleep and meal times to meet the new time zone before traveling. Staying hydrated while traveling and avoiding alcohol during flights may also make sleeping easier.

Managing Food Triggers Without Altering Your Diet

Perhaps my favorite non-diet companion to the low-FODMAP diet is the use of digestive enzyme supplementation. Digestive enzymes are proteins that act on food to break it down to its simplest, digestible form and otherwise have no impact on the body whatsoever. If you are not deficient in the enzyme contained in your supplement, then your body will digest the enzyme like any other protein. If you take a digestive enzyme supplement and you are deficient in that enzyme, or you take a digestive enzyme that our bodies don't make, your body will use it to break down that food and limit triggering IBS symptoms. Digestive enzyme supplementation can improve your experience with food and liberalize your diet by allowing you to eat high-FODMAP foods without consequence. There are a number of digestive enzymes that have been shown to be highly effective for those with IBS.

Lactose

Lactose is the disaccharide found in dairy products. Our bodies make lactase, the enzyme that breaks down lactose into glucose and galactose, but it is very common for people not to produce enough lactose as they age or if they have had inflammation or damage to their small intestine. As we discussed in Chapter 4, you can be tested for lactose intolerance via a breath test, but if you think you are intolerant to lactose, you can experiment by using a lactase enzyme supplement with meals that contain dairy.

To start, take 9,000 units just before or with your first bite. Lactase enzymes are available in pill and chewable forms. Brands will differ on dosage, so read the package in order to take enough to cover your meal. Lactase supplementation will last about 30 minutes, so if you are out to eat and have cheese with your appetizer and ice cream for dessert, you will most likely need a second dose with dessert. You cannot overdose on lactase supplementation. As mentioned before, enzymes are proteins and will be broken down by the body just like the protein in chicken and nuts if not used to break down lactose.

Alpha-Galactosidase

Alpha-galactosidase is the enzyme that breaks down some carbohydrates like the ones found in galacto-oligosaccharides (or in the oligosaccharide group of FODMAPs). The enzyme occurs naturally in the body but not in the amount that anyone needs to fully break the carbohydrates down, therefore microbes will ferment them and produce gas. The most common example of a carbohydrate that needs alpha-galactosidase to break it down is beans. You know the familiar childhood limerick about beans being good for your heart and what happens when you eat them? It's the truth! Unfortunately for those with IBS, that gas formation can lead to bloating, distension, and excess, odorous gas.

There are a number of enzyme supplements that contain alpha-galactosidase. The effective dose is 300 units and you can take up to 1,200 units at a meal (although that's probably not necessary), and they are available in pills and melts. A well-known brand in the U.S. contains mannitol, a polyol, but not in an amount that is high-FODMAP so it is safe to use even if polyol-containing foods trigger your IBS symptoms.

Other Enzymes with Promising Outcomes

Glucose isomerase is an enzyme that converts fructose into glucose. Remember that to absorb fructose, you need glucose as a partner, but glucose doesn't need any partners as it is easily absorbed on its own for those who don't have insulin sensitivity or diabetes. Glucose isomerase has been packaged as an enzyme supplement for those with excess fructose intolerance. In theory, this is a good idea since fructose is a simple sugar and can't be broken down further, and there is some anecdotal evidence of beneficial outcomes from its use. However, there is no research supporting that it works for the masses. There is no harm in trying it, though it may not work for you.

Fructan hydrolase is an enzyme recently created to break down fructans like the ones found in garlic and onions and wheat. This is a proprietary enzyme available in only one brand of supplements. This enzyme is sprinkled and mixed into your food just before eating. In one study conducted by the company that created it, 90 percent of fructans in the food were broken down within 30 minutes of its use before consuming it (Ochoa et al., 2022). There is no need to wait the 30 minutes—the enzyme will work while on your food and when it enters your digestive system upon eating. The data on this enzyme is promising, though we need more independent research to confirm its effectiveness for the masses. Like other enzymes, it is safe to take and will be digested as a protein if unused.

Inulase is an enzyme touted to break down inulin, a fructan. There are two forms of it, endo-inulase and exo-inulase, and each plays a different role in the breakdown of fructans. While products on the market that contain both endo- and exo-inulase purport to break down fructans, there is no research available on any form of inulase used for FODMAP breakdown. The current research on inulase focuses on how it breaks down fructans to create high-fructose corn syrup in the food industry but not in the body.

Missing from this list are enzymes that break down polyols or sugar alcohols and that's because they do not exist. Manufacturers are working on a solution to this, but in the meantime, if you have an intolerance to polyols, you will need to limit your portions or avoid them.

You can take dietary enzymes with the low-FODMAP diet or instead of the low-FODMAP diet. If you are a candidate for the low-FODMAP diet and have been through the elimination phase and the reintroduction phase, you now know what your trigger foods are. To further liberalize your diet, you can reintroduce your trigger foods again, but this time while using a digestive enzyme supplement with your trial. For instance, if beans are a trigger for you, you can take alpha-galactosidase with your first bite of your beans and keep track of any symptoms throughout the day. You do not need to do a three-day trial while using the digestive enzymes—they should work on your first try. Remember that food is not just made up of one nutrient or component and if you do have symptoms, it might be from something else you ate. Remember to also pay attention to your stress levels and sleep habits surrounding the day of the trial as IBS symptoms can have numerous triggers.

If you are not a candidate for the low-FODMAP diet, you can use digestive enzymes in two ways. The first is to use them with every meal so that you don't need to consider what is in your food before eating it. This is especially helpful for those with disordered eating and eating disorders. However, if you choose to use digestive enzymes in this way, remember that there are only enzymes available for oligosaccharides, disaccharides, and monosaccharides, and *not* for polyols.

The other way to use enzymes without the low-FODMAP diet is to consider what FODMAPs might be in your food and take the enzyme specific to that FODMAP. For instance, if you are having a bean and cheese taco, you could take lactase and alpha-galactosidase, but if you are having yogurt, you would take only lactase.

Managing Constipation and Slow Motility

There might be a number of causes driving constipation and slow motility. We know the roles that stress, poor sleep, and food play in IBS management, but for those with motility issues, the driving force may be a lack of driving force. In other words, constipation can be due to weak muscles in the pelvic floor that are not strong enough to move bowels without straining. Or your constipation can be due to other diagnoses that damage connective tissue (what our bowels are made of) and make our involuntary muscles and tissues throughout the intestines weaker, leading to less effective motility. In those cases, some behavior changes, medications, and supplements may alleviate constipation and get things moving again.

Fiber—Mushers and Pushers

There are two types of fiber in our food supply and both play a role in relieving constipation. They are soluble fiber and insoluble fiber, or as I tell my clients, *mushers* and *pushers*. Soluble fiber sources are your mushers. Soluble fiber is like a sponge—it soaks up water and turns into a gel-like "mush" in your digestive system. It works to soften your stool, making it easier to pass through your intestines. This type of fiber slows down digestion and can help with issues like diarrhea because it absorbs extra water, creating a more solid stool. Examples of foods high in soluble fiber include oats, chia seeds, the flesh of apples, and squash.

Insoluble fiber is like the broom of your digestive system. It doesn't dissolve in water; instead, it stays mostly intact as it moves through your gut. This type of fiber sweeps through your gut, causing mucus to be excreted, which helps to lubricate your stool, and pushes waste along for easier movement. Insoluble fiber speeds up digestion, which is especially helpful if things are feeling stuck. Examples of foods high in insoluble fiber include whole grains like whole wheat, nuts, the skin and seeds of vegetables, and leafy greens.

Your gut loves a balance of both mushers and pushers because they keep your digestive system running smoothly. When you have constipation, having soluble fiber-rich foods can help to move things along, especially if you experience incomplete evacuations. However, eating enough of both types of fiber will help to keep your stool soft as well as moving along.

Fiber Supplementation

If getting fiber from your diet isn't enough, you have the option to use a fiber supplement. Supplements are available in powders and pills. Powdered fiber supplements, mixed into tepid or cold water, might be flavored or unflavored. If you need more insoluble fiber to push things along and encourage complete evacuations, you might want to try calcium polycarbophil. If you have hard stool and would like to soften it using a fiber supplement, a good choice is psyllium. Make sure to drink adequate amounts of fluid so that soluble fiber supplements can absorb water in the gut and insoluble fiber will have something to push along and out.

Laxatives

When you have constipation-predominant IBS, your digestive system moves slowly, making it hard to go to the bathroom. Laxatives are medications that can remedy that. There are two common types used for IBS-C: osmotic laxatives and stimulant laxatives.

Osmotic Laxatives: The "Water Pullers"

Osmotic laxatives work by pulling water into your intestines. The water in your gut softens your stool and makes it easier to pass. They work somewhat like soluble fiber. Osmotic laxatives are gentle on your system and take a while to work so they won't trigger urgency to move your bowels. Examples of osmotic laxatives include polyethylene glycol and lactulose.

Stimulant Laxatives: The "Gut Kick-Starters"

Stimulant laxatives give your intestines a little nudge—or more like a kick—to get them moving. They irritate the lining of your gut to help the muscles contract, which pushes the stool out faster. Stimulant laxatives are stronger than the osmotic types and work more quickly. When osmotic laxatives don't work or don't work on their own, adding in a stimulant laxative can get things moving. Examples of stimulant laxatives include senna and bisacodyl.

There are a few downsides to stimulant laxatives. First, they can cause cramping, which can be uncomfortable in addition to the negative sensations that constipation already causes. Second, using them regularly can lead to your intestines relying on them to function. Third, there is a risk of misuse of stimulant laxatives among those with eating disorders, so if you have been diagnosed with an eating disorder or you have disordered eating tendencies, it's best to avoid them.

Laxative use is not a long-term solution. If you rely on them too often, your symptoms may get worse over time. It's important to talk to your healthcare provider about incorporating laxative use into your dietary changes, medication, and other supplementation as part of your toolbox instead of as your only tool.

A Few Other Movement Makers

Magnesium

Magnesium, a mineral found in many foods, works like a gentle helper for your intestines as an osmotic laxative via supplementation.

It draws water into your gut and relaxes the muscles in your digestive tract to make it easier for stool to pass. There are a few forms of magnesium available. Magnesium citrate is the version used in a number of colonoscopy preparations and it is the strongest version. Magnesium oxide is gentler and safe to use regularly. I often suggest to my clients to take their dose all at once in the evening since some people get drowsy at higher doses of magnesium. Speak with your healthcare provider to determine the dose that will work best for you.

Stool Softeners

Stool softeners add moisture to stool by drawing in water like an osmotic laxative. If you tend to strain when you move your bowels, a stool softener like docusate sodium can help without making things move faster. They are a good tool for people who have pain or discomfort while pooping and whose stool is a hard consistency.

Kiwifruit Kiwi has been studied by researchers in, where else, New Zealand, the home of the kiwifruit, to support constipation management. Eating two kiwis a day has been shown to reduce constipation and improve gut motility without a laxative effect. The fruit can be eaten with or without the skin, whole or in a smoothie. Kiwi also contains soluble fiber that is low in FODMAPs so it can be added to your toolbox while on the low-FODMAP diet elimination phase.

Prunes If you are of a certain generation, this might be the only tool you know of to help with constipation. Prunes are dried plums and they are known for their ability to help with getting things moving. They contain sorbitol, a polyol and a sugar alcohol that acts by pulling water into the intestines and softening stool. They also contain both soluble and insoluble fiber. In a recent study, a test group consumed 12 prunes a day. Another test group consumed eight ounces of prune juice and reaped the same benefits. If 12 prunes sounds like a lot, start with two a day and increase your intake until you find your magic number. Prunes can have a laxative effect and cause cramping, so if they upset your system more than they help, use a different tool.

Toileting Regimen

A toileting regimen is a group of behaviors that make moving your bowels a daily habit and so is an effective tool. Creating your own regimen can help if you are not in tune with your bodily cues or don't notice when you have an early sensation to move your bowels.

Start by drinking a hot or warm beverage in the mornings as this can trigger the *gastrocolic reflex*. This is when the GI system awakens and is stimulated by the intake of food or fluid to make room for what is entering the system by moving everything down toward the exit. In those with IBS-D, the gastrocolic reflex can be overstimulated and when something is consumed, it can signal the bowels to empty every time (that pesky drama queen, visceral hypersensitivity, at work again). For those with constipation, however, hot or warm liquid can awaken that sleepy system. Taking a fiber supplement with your warm beverage or in addition in a cold beverage or smoothie can also be part of your toileting regimen and will help to create the habit of taking the fiber supplement daily.

Toileting positioning and sitting on the toilet daily is part of the regimen. Positioning your knees higher than your hips using a stool, books, or yoga blocks allows your pelvic floor to relax and helps with elimination. If you don't have a stool or other leg-raising equipment, you can mimic the body position by putting your elbows on your thighs and your chin in your hands, if this is accessible to you. Spend no more than five to ten minutes sitting without actively or continuously pushing or straining. If nothing passes during that time, you can leave the bathroom. If, at another time during the day, you sense a signal to go, prioritize that signal and head to the bathroom. If you don't go when you feel the signal and hold it in to either go at a more convenient time or wait until you get home, water in your stool might be drawn out, making the stool hard and leading to an exacerbation of your symptoms later on.

Over time, a toileting regimen creates a moment of mindfulness to listen to and learn your cues to move your bowels. Those with slow motility may not feel signals daily. In those cases, a motility aid in the form of medication or a supplement may help.

Prescription Medications

As a registered dietitian, it is not within my scope of practice to recommend or prescribe medications for any diagnosis, including IBS. There are, however, a number of medications on the market that target constipation in different ways. These are typically used in conjunction with other constipation remedies and are often prescribed when other tools are ineffective or cease to work. Talk with your physician to see if a prescription drug aimed at constipation could help you to better manage your IBS.

Secretagogues

Secretagogues help draw water into the intestines and make it easier for stool to move through. Although helpful, it might be difficult to have a formed bowel movement when first starting on these drugs. Examples include linaclotide, plecanatide, and lubiprostone.

Serotonin Type-4 Receptor Agonists (5-HT4 Agonists)

These speed up the movement of food through the digestive system and increase fluid in the intestines. They are used for more severe cases of IBS-C. They can cause mild cramping because they trigger motility. Examples include prucalopride and tegaserod.

Prescription-Strength Osmotic Laxatives

When the over-the-counter laxatives aren't working, higher doses and stronger medications may be what you need. They also work like over-the-counter osmotic laxatives by pulling water into the intestines, softening stool, and making it easier to pass. As with other laxatives, they may not be appropriate for everyday use. Consult with your prescribing physician for dosing and frequency. Examples of prescription-strength osmotic laxatives include lactulose and polyethylene glycol 3350.

Peripherally Acting Mu-Opioid Receptor Antagonists (PAMORAs)

If you have pain that is managed by opioids, you might find that they exacerbate your constipation from IBS. PAMORAs are prescribed when constipation is caused by opioid medications. They work by blocking opioids from affecting the gut without interfering with the pain relief they provide. In my practice, I have seen clients who are not on opioids but are prescribed these drugs for hard-to-treat constipation due to slow motility. Examples include methylnaltrexone and naloxegol.

Managing Diarrhea and Fast Motility

If you have IBS with diarrhea, you are among those whose digestive system moves too quickly. Urgency to move your bowels along with frequent trips to the bathroom can have a significant impact on quality of life. There are many strategies and treatments to help slow things down and reduce symptoms. These can be used alone or in conjunction with one another to create your trigger management toolbox.

Fiber and Fiber Supplements

Fiber isn't just for constipation, it can help with diarrhea too. Besides softening stool, soluble fiber—aka the "mushers"—absorbs water in your gut and helps thicken stools. This can reduce the urgency and frequency of diarrhea and help with creating formed bowel movements. Including food sources like bananas, oats, and squash in your diet may help, but fiber supplementation may be needed if you are not able to get adequate fiber through eating alone.

Fiber supplementation for loose stools includes psyllium husk; the fiber that softens stool in those with constipation also helps to form stool in those with diarrhea. Sounds like magic, but it's simply soluble fiber forming a gelatinous substance that works for both IBS types. Other sources of soluble fiber for managing diarrhea include methylcellulose, partially hydrolyzed guar gum, acacia fiber, and wheat dextrin. Wheat dextrin does not contain FODMAPs (and can be gluten-free) so it will not trigger someone with a fructan intolerance or those with a gluten sensitivity or celiac disease, but only if it is labeled gluten-free.

Over-the-Counter Medication for Diarrhea and Fast Motility

There are some over-the-counter medications that can help to slow motility and reduce the accompanying cramping. Antispasmodics calm the muscles of your intestines to reduce cramping and spasms that can lead to diarrhea. They also act as a pain reliever. The most effective over-the-counter version is enteric-coated peppermint oil. Enteric-coated means that the capsule will not open from being exposed to stomach acid and will release its contents when it reaches the small intestine. Taking a capsule 30 minutes before each meal can prevent urgency after meals. They can be taken three times a day to prevent urgency and to slow motility, or used when needed to relieve pain from cramping in the intestines.

Antidiarrheal medications can also slow down gut motility and firm up stools. They are a good tool for short-term use such as before a big event or while traveling, but they may also be recommended by your doctor for everyday use. Examples include loperamide and bismuth subsalicylate. In addition to acting as an antidiarrheal, bismuth subsalicylate coats the stomach and intestines, reducing inflammation and irritation. It also has mild antibacterial properties that can target harmful gut bacteria and reduce diarrhea. In some cases, it can help reduce gas and bloating.

Prescription Medications for Diarrhea and Fast Motility

When the over-the-counter tools are not doing the trick, speak with your doctor about your options for prescription medications that may be more effective in reducing urgency and forming stool. There are prescription-strength antispasmodics that can be taken every day or just when needed. Examples include dicyclomine, hyoscyamine, and eluxadoline. Dicyclomine is taken in pill form while hyoscyamine is placed under the tongue and works very quickly to stop spasms. Eluxadoline can be taken up to two times a day with food but should not be taken more often because it is a controlled substance and can lead to misuse or dependence.

Low-dose tricyclic antidepressants (TCAs) can also reduce pain and lead to formed stool. Examples include amitriptyline and duloxetine. They work by affecting serotonin, a chemical in the brain and gut that helps control digestion, mood, and pain signals. In people with IBS-D, TCAs reduce the amount of serotonin in the gut, which slows down digestion and decreases diarrhea. They also calm the nerves in the gut, which can reduce pain and cramping. Even though these drugs are referred to as "antidepressants," the dose used to manage IBS symptoms is much lower than the dose used to treat depression.

Managing Gas, Bloating, and Distension

Perhaps the most frustrating symptoms to manage are excess gas, bloating, and distension. These symptoms develop for many reasons, such as trapped gas, slow digestion, imbalances in gut bacteria, and visceral hypersensitivity. Fortunately, there are a few tools at your disposal to experiment with and see if they bring you relief.

Simethicone is an over-the-counter medication that helps break up gas bubbles in the stomach and intestines, making it easier to pass gas. It doesn't prevent gas from forming but can provide quick relief from bloating and discomfort caused by trapped gas. It's available in chewable form and melts and is safe to take numerous times throughout the day, if needed. It can also be taken prior to meals to reduce the formation of large gas bubbles.

STW 5

STW 5 is a natural herbal remedy made from a blend of plants and herbs, such as chamomile, peppermint, and caraway. It can help reduce bloating by relaxing the muscles in your digestive tract and improving how food and gas move through your system. It also has anti-inflammatory properties, which can calm an irritated gut. In 2023, this product was reformulated due to a rare side effect of liver injury. The manufacturer has since removed three herbs and the remaining six show promise of effectiveness without risky side effects.

Prebiotic Fiber Supplementation

Prebiotic fibers, such as partially hydrolyzed guar gum (PHGG), can help support the growth of beneficial gut bacteria. Prebiotic fiber acts as a fertilizer for the microbiome, allowing strains and colonies of microbes to feed off it if they are in need of balance. This balance of bacteria can reduce bloating and gas over time. It's important to start with small amounts of prebiotic fiber and increase gradually, as introducing too much too quickly can exacerbate bloating. Prebiotics are found in food, but most of them are high in FODMAPs. PHGG is slow to ferment and can be used regularly. If, after 30 days, you do not see an improvement in symptoms, you do not need to continue with it. If you do find that your gas, bloating, and distension have abated, you can take prebiotics daily or take them for 30 days intermittently with a 30-day break.

Belly Massage

An abdominal massage can help relieve gas and bloating by physically pushing it along. Massage can stimulate your intestines, encouraging trapped gas to pass more easily and reduce bloating. It's easy to do at home and many people find it relaxing. You can do it in any position but it's probably most comfortable if you are lying down. Imagine your large intestine is an upside-down U. Using the flat part of your fingers, apply gentle but firm pressure to the bottom right side of your belly. Working in small, circular motions, slowly move up your right side, across your belly just below your ribs to the left side, then down the left side. Once you complete the upside-down U, you can continue the massage from the left side even with your left hip and move toward the midline and stop. This massage can be repeated a few times in a row. Taking slow, deep breaths as you work will help with relaxation.

The use of a heating pad or a warm compress before, after, or instead of an abdominal massage can offer additional relaxation and the release of trapped gas. Use it for no more than 20 minutes at a time and be mindful of your heat settings so that you don't burn your skin.

Avoiding Straws

Using drinking straws can worsen gas and bloating in people with IBS because straws increase the amount of air you swallow while drinking. This swallowed air, called aerophagia, can enter the digestive tract and lead to excess gas, bloating, and distension. If you suffer from trapped gas, avoid straws whenever possible and drink directly from the cup or glass.

Behavioral Changes for Managing IBS

In addition to medication and supplements, there are simple, non-diet behavioral changes you can make to reduce symptoms and improve your quality of life. These strategies involve approaching symptom management with compassion.

Loose Clothing

Tight clothing, especially around your stomach, can put pressure on your abdomen and make bloating, gas, and cramping feel worse. In some cases, tight clothing can trigger bloating and distension, thanks to visceral hypersensitivity. Wearing loose-fitting clothes, such as stretchy pants or relaxed tops, can reduce unnecessary stress on your digestive system while giving your body space to expand without discomfort when you do experience symptoms.

Gentle Movement

Light physical activity, like walking, stretching, or yoga, can help move gas through your intestines and improve digestion. Exercise also stimulates the release of endorphins, which are natural chemicals that make you feel good and can help reduce stress—a major trigger for IBS symptoms. Listen to your body and do what feels good to you. No need to keep up with the latest workout trends if they lead to more IBS discomfort.

Mindful Eating

Mindful eating is about paying attention while you eat. Eat slowly, chew your food thoroughly, and avoid distractions that keep you from being mindful, like watching TV or scrolling on your phone during meals. This habit can reduce the amount of air you swallow and help prevent bloating and discomfort. Mindful eating also helps you tune into your hunger and fullness signals, which can prevent eating past fullness and subsequently triggering GI discomfort.

Stress Management

Everyone experiences stress. Even if stress is not your main IBS trigger, techniques like deep breathing, meditation, or progressive muscle relaxation can calm your nervous system and reduce the impact of stress on your gut from existing in our world. Setting aside just five to ten minutes a day for relaxation can be effective.

Consistent Routines

Keeping a regular daily routine, especially for eating and sleeping, can help regulate your body's internal clock and improve digestion. Try to eat regularly and adequately, about every three to four hours, as our digestive tract is a series of muscles and appreciates being used throughout the day to best function. Aiming for a full night's rest every evening that begins and ends around the same time keeps your circadian rhythm happy, which keeps your digestion and motility running smoothly.

Bathroom Habits

When you need to use the bathroom, don't hold it in as this can lead to constipation or other issues. If you experience urgency, make adjustments to your schedule, giving yourself time to move your bowels as often as you need to before starting your day or leaving the house.

By making these small, non-diet changes, you can take control of your IBS symptoms and improve how you feel every day. These steps, combined with other treatments, will help you to create your toolbox of IBS symptom managers. Approach the process of filling your toolbox with compassion and curiosity. If something doesn't work for you, chances are there is another option or combination of options that will. It bears repeating that a log will help you to see what offers improvement, even if it's slow to come. If you need help building your toolbox, always reach out to your healthcare practitioners for guidance.

Non-Diet Interventions That Need More Research

Managing IBS often involves exploring a variety of treatments, but you shouldn't be the guinea pig in the experiment (unless you have actually consented to taking part in a research study). Some non-diet approaches to managing IBS might show promise but require more research to confirm their effectiveness, and some have the research but are still being recommended despite their ineffectiveness. If you choose to explore any of these, you do so at your own risk.

Acupuncture

Acupuncture is an ancient practice where thin needles are inserted into specific points on the body to stimulate nerves and promote healing. Some studies suggest acupuncture may help reduce IBS symptoms like pain and bloating, possibly by calming the nervous system or improving gut motility. However, these studies often have small sample sizes, making it difficult to know if the results apply to larger groups of people. Additionally, the placebo effect is a concern since IBS symptoms are highly influenced by psychological factors. While some people with IBS report benefits, there are challenges with studying acupuncture due to the inability to form a control group. More well-designed research is needed to confirm its effectiveness for IBS management. However, using acupuncture, delivered by a trained practitioner, will not cause you harm and should not trigger symptoms.

Yoga

Yoga combines gentle movement, breathing exercises, and mindfulness, which could be helpful for people with IBS by calming the gut–brain axis, thereby reducing stress and improving gut motility. A few small studies show that yoga may alleviate symptoms like abdominal pain, diarrhea, or constipation. However, these studies often lack control groups or follow participants for a short period only. While yoga is safe and has benefits for overall health, it's unclear whether it has a specific and measurable impact on IBS.

Probiotics

You may have noticed that probiotics were not recommended as an option for your toolbox. Probiotics are live bacteria and yeast that are thought to improve gut health. Some studies suggest they may help with IBS symptoms like bloating, gas, and irregular bowel movements by restoring balance in the gut microbiome. As vast as the research is, the benefits are just not there. We do not yet know enough about our diverse microbiome to really understand what microbes need partner microbes to provide a beneficial outcome, or what microbes need the byproducts of other microbes in order to function properly. When we supplement our microbiome with strains of microbes, we may be helping, but we may be doing nothing at all. There is also no regulation on probiotic supplements so the amount of live bacteria and yeast listed on the label may not be the same amount as when you buy it or start taking it. Probiotics are seen as safe for people with IBS, but in the long run you might just be wasting money by taking them.

Herbal Remedies

Natural or holistic remedies are often explored as a way to manage IBS symptoms without medication, but the evidence for their effectiveness is mixed or not strong enough to make clear recommendations. For example, aloe vera, which is sometimes used to relieve constipation, lacks consistent evidence to prove it works for IBS, and it may even cause diarrhea in some people. St. John's Wort, which is commonly used for depression, does not appear to be effective for IBS symptoms when compared with antidepressant medications. It's important to consult with a healthcare provider before trying herbal remedies, as some can interact with your prescription medications or have side effects.

Fecal Microbiota Transplantation (FMT)

FMT involves transferring stool from a healthy donor into the gut of someone with an imbalanced microbiome. It has shown success in treating certain conditions like *Clostridioides difficile* infections and is being explored for IBS. Back when I was diagnosed, FMT was not well known. I was curious about it and spoke with my doctor about using it to heal my gut after my *C. diff* infection was gone. At that time, it was not legal for medical doctors to perform FMT unless there was active *C. diff* in the gut (although there were some alternative practitioners doing it and even some people doing it themselves). After some time passed and more research was done, no significant benefit was seen for people with IBS. There are some risks involved, including the variability in donor stool, so I would strongly suggest not taking this on yourself and speaking with your healthcare provider about the most up-to-date research.

For many of these interventions, the lack of large, well-designed studies is a major barrier to understanding their effectiveness. Small sample sizes, short follow-up periods, and inconsistent methodologies make it difficult to compare results across studies. Additionally, IBS is a complex condition influenced by multiple factors—what works for one person may not work for another. Stick with what is proven to be safe and effective when building your symptom management toolbox.

8
Living Well with IBS

Living with irritable bowel syndrome can be challenging, but it doesn't have to control your life. With the right tools, strategies, and mindset, you can navigate everyday situations, advocate for your needs, and live a fulfilling life. Now that you have the tools for managing your IBS, you can focus on practical tips for managing the logistical and emotional aspects of living with a chronic disease, from finding a bathroom in a hurry to traveling with confidence. My hope for you is that whether you are vacationing, working with your healthcare providers, or simply trying to enjoy a day out, you will feel in charge of your IBS despite the challenges it brings.

Creating Your Symptom Management Toolbox

In the last few chapters, we reviewed dietary interventions as well as behavioral changes, medications, supplements, and other non-diet tools to manage your IBS. Not all of these tools will work for you, but in order to know what will, you will need to begin experimenting. Keep a detailed daily log that includes:

- what you eat
- your symptoms
- your bathroom habits
- your sleep habits
- your stress levels.

This helps to pinpoint whether you are being triggered by food, poor sleep, or stress. Approach this information with as much objectiveness as you can muster. Apply a tool to alleviate the symptom or the cause and keep track of what works for you and what might not be effective. As you make your way through all of the tools, you will be adding to your toolbox. The goal is to have one or two remedies for each of your symptoms. This may mean working with your gastroenterologist to determine what prescription medications are helpful and which provide no relief, and working with a registered dietitian to determine what dietary intervention will be safe and effective for you.

Your symptom management toolbox should not turn into a dusty old container with rusty bits of ineffective gadgets that take up space. If an intervention no longer works for you, remove it from your toolbox. This may mean discontinuing a medication or adding a food to your "unsuccessful reintroduction" list. Doing so creates space for you to try another intervention and determine whether it is effective enough to be the shiny new gizmo in your toolbox. Your toolbox might be ever-changing, or it might stay the same for a long time. Either way, it's always a good idea to check in with yourself and see how you are feeling and if your toolbox could use a refresh.

Navigating Public Spaces: Finding a Bathroom

One of the saddest things I hear from clients is that they no longer leave the house unless they have to. The fear of not finding a restroom in time should they need one keeps them close to home, missing out on social opportunities with friends and family. Sometimes the fear is real due to urgency and the experience of fecal incontinence that can leave you traumatized, especially if it has happened in a public place. For some, though, the anxiety of "what if" is enough to stop even the formerly most adventurous traveler. With some practice, though, you can develop some resilience in the face of bathroom anxiety.

Planning ahead is the first step in feeling comfortable moving throughout the world with IBS. Certainly, use the tools from your toolbox to manage symptoms the best you can so that you don't experience fecal incontinence or painful urgency away from home, and to minimize symptoms when flares arise. When venturing out, pack extra meds in case you have symptoms. You might also want to take a change of underwear and wipes should you have an accident.

Knowing the layout of the places you are going, like a mall or a park, and where in those spaces the bathrooms are located, can be as easy as looking at a map online before leaving home. If you are exploring a city or running errands, it can be helpful to have a restroom locator app on your smartphone. There are a number of them available, mostly covering city areas. If you are in a more rural location, consider searching online for gas stations, rest stops, fast-food restaurants, book stores, and libraries along your route where bathrooms are available for public use without being expected to make a purchase.

One item that I suggest my clients with bathroom anxiety keep in their vehicles is a camping toilet. These are quick to set up or keep assembled and stored in your car. They can be used in a vehicle that has space to put it on the floor in the back seat, in the rear section of an SUV, or carried outside of the car to a wooded area for outdoor privacy. Keep toilet paper or wipes with you in case the need arises when you can't find a convenient place to stop. Over the years, I have found that clients who keep a camping toilet in their car have reduced anxiety from fear of not finding a restroom in time, even if they have never had to use it. One client experienced multiple incidences of fecal incontinence while driving. He had just a ten-minute commute to work from his home and would use the restroom before leaving the house and make a stop along the way almost every day. Once the camping toilet was in his car, he no longer needed to stop on the way to work, and he had no more episodes of fecal incontinence. It's amazing how a piece of camping equipment can reduce anxiety and alleviate IBS symptoms.

Traveling with IBS

Planes, trains, and automobile travel all come with their own set of challenges for people with all IBS subtypes. Preparing ahead is key to reducing anxiety and symptoms just as it is with local travel.

Planes

When we fly, the cabin is pressurized to mimic being at 10,000 feet above sea level even though we fly around 30,000 feet above sea level. However, the vast majority of us do not live our lives at 10,000 feet above sea level; I'm at 174 feet in my neighborhood. Being that high in the sky can significantly impact the body in several ways.

As altitude increases, the pressure decreases, causing gases in the body to expand. This can lead to increased gas in the intestines, which can worsen bloating and discomfort. This expanded gas can cause cramping, a feeling of fullness, and increased urgency to use the restroom. A change in air pressure can impact the way your gastrointestinal system moves food and gas through the digestive tract, sometimes slowing it down. Add low humidity to the change in pressure and you might experience an exacerbation of symptoms like constipation for those with IBS-C. Make sure to stay well hydrated before, during, and after flying to reduce the likelihood of being constipated for days after your flight. It is also helpful to move about the plane (when it is safe to do so) by walking and stretching to encourage motility.

If you have IBS-D, flying can add a layer of stress that can impact visceral hypersensitivity and trigger urgency. The added anxiety of being confined and not having immediate access to a bathroom can make symptoms worse. If you use antispasmodics on occasion, then before you fly would be a good occasion to take them. If you take them regularly, make sure to stay on your schedule, even with a time change, until you have adjusted. Make one last trip to the restroom in the airport to ease your mind before boarding.

You might have noticed that flying also increases gas buildup in your gut—another fun side effect from the change in cabin pressure. Avoiding carbonated beverages on the day of your trip and while in the air will minimize the build-up of excess gas in the system. Taking simethicone before take-off can help break down those impending gas bubbles into smaller and more easily passable bubbles.

Changes to eating patterns such as eating at irregular times, not eating adequately at meals, or not having access to safe foods can also upset digestion. If food is a trigger for you, avoid eating your trigger foods the day before and the day of your flight. Instead, focus on what you might bring with you for a day of travel and what will be available to you at the airport and on the flight so that you can plan accordingly. You can contact the airline to request special meals (if meals are served on your flight) to meet your needs. If they are not able to accommodate you—most airlines will have options for passengers with food allergies, such as a nut-free meal, but they don't offer low-FODMAP meals—make sure you pack food to support your needs for the duration of the trip.

Even before arriving at the airport, make sure to pack essentials: Bring any medications, low-FODMAP snacks, and other comfort items to manage symptoms during the flight. Wireless, rechargeable heating pads can be a great tool to carry with you to help keep your belly relaxed and calm. Although flying can pose challenges for those with IBS, it's possible to minimize discomfort and enjoy your journey with just a little preparation and awareness.

Trains

While traveling by train doesn't change the pressure within your body, you may still experience some of the anxiety that plane travelers do. Prepare by packing an IBS-friendly travel kit complete with low-FODMAP meals and snacks, medications, and heating pad, know where the restrooms are located in the train terminal prior to leaving, and where to find restrooms once you board. You may want to pack tissues or wipes in case those restrooms are not well stocked. If you are booking an overnight passage on a train, consider an aisle seat near the restroom so that you don't have to climb over a fellow passenger and don't have far to go in case of a personal emergency.

Sitting on a train is a great time to practice relaxation techniques like deep breathing and meditation. Staying relaxed and calm will not only help to manage any symptoms should they arise but will also help manage anxiety should unexpected delays occur.

Automobiles

Taking a long trip by car may seem less limiting to your access to a restroom or proper nutrition than by plane or train, but it's quite common that people with IBS will opt to skip meals and beverages on long rides to avoid experiencing urgency on unfamiliar roads. With a little planning, you can locate rest stops prior to the trip and places to grab a meal or a snack. Don't forget about that camping toilet now located in the back of your car for just-in-case moments. Packing a cooler full of low-FODMAP foods can be a good idea. To avoid constipation, make sure to drink plenty of fluids and plan to make stops to urinate. Eating at regular intervals with adequate intake will keep your system running smoothly so that you can enjoy a symptom-free time both while on your journey and when you reach your destination.

Eating Out

Eating out, whether at a restaurant or at a loved one's home, can feel stressful when you have IBS. Worrying about food triggers, finding options that won't upset your stomach, and explaining your dietary needs to others can make social gatherings anxiety-provoking. However, with a little planning and self-advocacy, you can enjoy meals outside of your home while minimizing discomfort, reducing the risk of triggering symptoms, and having the opportunity to eat when you are hungry.

When dining at a restaurant, planning ahead is key. Many restaurants post their menus online, making it easier to see what your options are before arriving. If you are not sure about the ingredients in a dish, contact the restaurant and ask. The purveyors want you to dine with them and will typically make substitutions so that you have an enjoyable experience in their establishment. If you don't have the time to plan, you can ask questions when you are seated by speaking with your server. If they don't know the answers, politely ask to speak to the manager or chef to ensure that what you order is in line with your dietary needs. If you are not comfortable asking questions, then choose simple meals that contain grilled proteins, steamed vegetables, and gluten-free starches like rice or potatoes. You can also use your toolbox and bring digestive enzymes with you to prevent symptoms from foods that might contain your trigger FODMAP ingredients.

Social gatherings at someone else's home can be tricky, but advocating for yourself in a polite and respectful way can help ensure you have a good time without stressing over food. You can begin by letting your host know about your dietary needs and asking what will be served so that you can plan accordingly. You might also offer to bring a dish to share that is free from your food triggers to ensure there will be something for you when the meal is served.

When hosting a gathering that includes food, remember that there might be others with food allergies, intolerances, or triggers that are different from yours. These guests would benefit from substitutions to what's being served too. Making a habit of asking your guests if they have dietary restrictions when you invite them gives those who are not so comfortable advocating for themselves the opportunity to speak up. I can't tell you how grateful I am when I go to an event and someone remembers my food intolerances and provides alternatives for me. I have also been in the situation where there is nothing to eat, and that can be quite uncomfortable, both for me and for the host.

Have a backup plan when going to events in case the food options don't suit your needs. You can eat a small meal before going to avoid being hungry if the options are limited. You can also pack some food and eat it when others are eating. Everything from granola bars to sandwiches can be stashed in a purse or a pocket so that you do not end up uncomfortably hungry.

When all else fails, try to remember that social gatherings are about more than food. Shift your focus to enjoying the company, conversations, and activities rather than worrying too much about what's on your plate. You will have the opportunity to eat again when the party is over.

Speaking up for your needs when eating out is all about preparation, communication, and confidence. With a little effort, you can enjoy meals with friends and family while keeping your IBS symptoms in check.

Advocating with Healthcare Practitioners

Living with IBS can be challenging, especially when you feel that your concerns aren't being taken seriously. Working with healthcare providers who understand your needs and goals is essential for managing your symptoms effectively. Learning how to ask for what you need and share your IBS story can help you get the care you deserve and create a successful partnership with your healthcare team.

Communicating Symptoms and Needs

One of the best ways to help your healthcare providers understand what you're going through is to share your log with them. The information you collect—what you are eating, your symptoms, when they happen, what your sleep is like, and how you were feeling—can help you and your practitioner find patterns and provide clear information. This can make it easier for them to figure out what might be triggering your symptoms and to suggest treatment options.

Using clear and specific language to describe your experiences is also helpful. Instead of saying, "My stomach hurts all the time," try being more specific. "I have sharp pain on my left side about 30 minutes after eating and it lasts for a few hours" is a clear and specific statement about the symptom duration, intensity, and possible cause. The more details you provide, the better your healthcare team can understand and thus offer effective support.

It's also helpful to arrive with a list of questions you have about your symptoms, treatments, or symptom management tools. Asking questions about what tests might be helpful or if there are other options for symptom management can get you the answers you seek. It's best to write a list so that you remember your questions and have a place to record the answers so that you can refer to them when making decisions about the options.

Navigating Difficult Conversations

Sometimes, conversations with your healthcare team members can be challenging. You might feel rushed, dismissed, or treated from a place of bias based on your race, gender, or size. If this happens, it's important to address dismissive comments by calmly explaining that you want to focus solely on managing your symptoms and be offered similar treatments that are offered to people of other races, genders, or size. Let them know what you have already tried and what has or hasn't worked for you by sharing your IBS story.

If you feel that your provider isn't listening or offering the right solutions, it's okay to seek a second opinion. Getting another perspective can help you find a healthcare professional who better understands your needs and offers treatment options that align with your goals.

Speaking up and setting boundaries doesn't mean arguing with your doctor; it means standing up for your health in a respectful and confident way. You have the right to feel heard and to receive equitable and respectful care.

Collaborative Care

Good healthcare should be a partnership between you and your provider. This approach, called patient-centered care, means that your doctor listens to your concerns, asks for consent before touching you and explains how you will be examined, provides you with options for care, respects your choices, and works with you to create a plan that fits your lifestyle. In collaborative care, both the patient and the healthcare provider have important roles to play.

As the patient, you will be expected to come prepared. Bring a list of questions and concerns. Honesty is an important factor in patient-centered care, even if that honesty is embarrassing; your provider's job is to help, not judge. Once your treatment plan is decided upon, it is your responsibility to follow through with the recommendations and provide feedback on what is or is not working for you. If you don't understand the treatment plan, ask questions so that when you leave the appointment you can take the necessary steps to enact the plan.

The role of the provider in patient-centered care is to actively listen to the patient and encourage shared decision-making. Throughout the appointment, your provider will offer evidence-based recommendations taken from research and clinical guidelines. These treatment options should align with your values and personal health goals. You may not normally feel like you and your doctor are "equals" during a healthcare visit, but in patient-centered care, you are teammates striving for the same goal. By working together and respecting each other's roles, the patient and the provider can build a strong partnership that leads to better symptom management and an improved quality of life. Remember, you are an active participant in your healthcare journey and your voice matters.

Addressing Weight Stigma

Weight stigma is when people are judged or treated unfairly because of their larger body size. It can happen anywhere—at work, in everyday interactions with friends and family, and at the doctor's office. Many people assume that being in a larger body automatically means someone is unhealthy or not taking care of themselves, but this is *not true*. The size of your body is not an indication of your health status, whether or not you exercise, or how much food you eat. Body size is largely determined by genetics. Yes, you can eat more than your body needs and put on weight, or restrict your intake and lose weight, but your body likes being in its natural state and will do what it can (send hunger signals, slow your metabolism to conserve energy stores) to bring you back to balance.

If you have ever dieted, you are most likely among the vast majority of people who regain the lost weight after going off the diet. You might have also experienced gaining back more weight than you initially lost. This is your body's way of preparing itself for the next time it experiences starvation. Fun fact: Your body doesn't know the difference between intentional weight-loss activities and unintended restriction, but it will prepare for them in the same way, beginning with slowing your metabolism, making it harder at every subsequent attempt to lose weight and drop those pounds.

Weight stigma can be harmful, especially for people with IBS, because it can get in the way of proper care and support. It can show up in subtle ways, for instance when healthcare providers assume that all of a patient's health problems are due to their weight, even when other factors may be causing symptoms. Some healthcare providers might focus only on weight loss as a solution rather than looking at other causes of symptoms. This can lead to unnecessary diets that don't actually help and may even make IBS worse. When your provider focuses solely on weight, they might overlook important treatments, such as stress management, medications, or research-based dietary interventions. This can leave people feeling frustrated, unheard, and still struggling with their symptoms. Their symptoms might even be worse after a visit where they experienced weight bias due to increased stress or starting a weight-loss diet that contains their food triggers. Not to mention, the awful experience might deter them from seeking additional care or a second opinion.

If you have experienced weight stigma in healthcare, it's important to know that you have the right to respectful and compassionate care no matter the size of your body. You can ask for weight-neutral approaches to treatment, meaning that your healthcare provider should focus on managing your symptoms rather than recommending weight loss as the first or only solution. Setting boundaries with your healthcare provider is another important step. If weight is repeatedly brought up as the main issue, you can kindly but firmly let them know that you would like to focus on symptom management and not discuss your weight. If you worry that you might experience weight bias, you can contact the doctor's office and ask them to make a note in your chart that your weight and weight loss are not discussed. If this is a first visit, you can add this request into the pre-appointment paperwork that you will most likely need to complete before being seen. Advocating for yourself in this way helps ensure that you receive the care you need while minimizing the harm from weight stigma.

Dealing with weight stigma can be challenging, but it's important to remember that your worth is not determined by the number on the scale. Seeking support from providers and communities that embrace body diversity can also help. Connecting with others who understand what you're going through can be empowering and reassuring. There are many weight-inclusive healthcare providers, social media groups, and support networks that can provide encouragement and resources to help you feel empowered when working with healthcare providers to ask for solutions that align with your values. By understanding weight stigma and the need for respectful care, you can take charge of managing your IBS in a way that feels supportive and empowering.

Building Resilience and Self-Compassion

A few years ago, I heard an upsetting statistic: In a study about the quality of life for people with chronic diseases, those with IBS scored lowest among others with chronic diseases including diabetes, reflux, depression, and dialysis-dependent end-stage kidney disease (Trindade et al., 2022). If you are not aware, people who are dialysis-dependent must have their kidneys flushed of waste and excess fluid for between three to five hours a few days each week, or three to four times a day for 90 minutes each session, depending on the type of dialysis. With all of that time spent managing their disease, they scored *higher* on quality-of-life scales than those with all subtypes of irritable bowel syndrome.

Living well with IBS not only includes taking charge of your symptoms by creating your toolbox and advocating for equitable care but also building resilience and self-compassion to deal with the moments that are not within your control. Having any chronic illness can be challenging, impacting both your body and your mind, but taking steps to create space for yourself when you are not feeling your best will make living with IBS more manageable, both physically and emotionally.

Let Go of Perfection

Even with all of the knowledge and tools you now possess, you will still have days when you don't feel your best. IBS is not a static disease; there will be some days that will be more difficult to manage than others, and no matter how vigilant you are, there will always be flares. The silver lining is that difficult days and flares are temporary. Allow yourself to experience these moments without judgment and use your tools to help you manage your discomfort until it passes.

Celebrate Small Wins

Every time you find a new food trigger or use a tool that effectively manages your symptoms, consider this a win. Focus on the positive steps you take, no matter how small. Did you try a new relaxation technique? Did you have a symptom-free day? Celebrate! Acknowledging these achievements can boost your confidence and well-being and be a reminder on rough days that you do have good days and they are just around the corner.

Create Support Systems

If 12–15 percent of the world's population has IBS, chances are you know someone who shares your diagnosis. Share your experiences with trusted friends and family members. Their understanding and encouragement can help alleviate feelings of isolation and stress. Connecting with others who share your diagnosis and understand what you are going through can also provide comfort and support. Online forums, educational websites, and your healthcare providers can offer valuable information and a sense of belonging. Imagine how great it would be to go out to eat with a group of new friends and not have to explain your menu choice or why you wanted to sit close to the bathroom. Knowing that everyone is in the same boat may also reduce anxiety when meeting up or eating out with your new connections.

A warning about those online forums: Some contain people who think that their experience outweighs research when it comes to the treatment options they have chosen. Before trying anything you hear about in these groups, reach out to your provider for guidance as to whether or not these options are safe, effective, and will be beneficial for you.

Stay Empowered

While you don't have complete control over your IBS, you can manage how you respond to it. Focus on what you can do, such as implementing dietary changes that are appropriate for you, experimenting with stress management techniques, and getting a good night's sleep on a regular basis. When something doesn't feel right, it's up to you to reach out to your healthcare team to seek support.

While there is no cure for IBS at this moment, keeping abreast of emerging treatments and symptom management tools can open up new avenues for managing your symptoms effectively and minimizing the effects of a flare. Research is being conducted all around the world. My hope for you is that one day soon, we will discover a cure for IBS and your pain and discomfort will be a thing of the past. Until that day, remember that you are not alone, and you are not powerless.

Through this book, you've gained the tools, knowledge, and strategies to better understand your body and take charge of your health. Whether it's identifying triggers, advocating for yourself in healthcare settings, or making choices that support your well-being, you now have the knowledge (and hopefully the confidence) to navigate life with IBS on your own terms. There will be ups and downs, but each step you take—no matter how small—is progress toward feeling better and living well. Whenever you feel uncertain or need a refresher, you can always turn back to this book as a trusted guide to help you stay on track. Trust yourself, be kind to your body, and know that with the right approach, support, and mindset, you can thrive. With patience and perseverance, your gut goals are within reach.

Acknowledgments

Four months after finishing this book, my editor asked if I wanted to include an acknowledgments page. I said "Yes!" without hesitation—and then immediately began to worry that I'd forget someone. I wrote this book by myself, but I didn't write it alone. It came to life because of the many people who taught me, worked alongside me, learned from me, supported me, and loved me. If I were to name each of you, it would take hundreds of pages. So instead, I offer this brief but heartfelt thank you to everyone who helped make this book possible.

To my children, Eli and Amelia—you are my heart. Eli, when you were little, you thought I sat around all day waiting for you to get home from school. You later discovered my job was, quite literally, talking about poop—and you became one of my biggest cheerleaders. Thank you for your wit, your curiosity, your sweetness, and your always special FaceTime calls. Amelia, from the moment you arrived, you've been a fierce, intuitive, and deeply loving presence in my life. You cheered me on every day while I wrote this book, and your encouragement carried me through some of the hardest chapters. Thank you, my loves.

I am endlessly grateful to my husband and lifelong friend, Mike—thank you for listening to endless poop talk (even at dinner), for reviewing contracts with your business brain, for celebrating my wins with me, and for your undying, unconditional love since camp. I love you.

Writing requires taking breaks and most of mine were unscheduled thanks to Willow "Beast" and Oakley "Captain Chaos" Rosen, the dynamic doggie duo that napped, fought, and played under my desk when they weren't begging for walks or my lunch.

My gratitude extends beyond the nucleus to my extended family—thank you for your unwavering support over the years. Mom, thank you for telling everyone (including the woman at Barnes & Noble) about my book, even before I finished writing it. To Jerry and Mel, I love you with all my heart. Thank you for being my bonus parents and checking in during my writing process. To my dad, z"l, I feel you around me every day. I know how proud you would be. And to my siblings, in-laws, nieces, and nephews—thank you for adapting meals to accommodate me, and for gluten-free bagels and matzah balls that said "we love you" in every bite.

When I first got sick, I struggled to leave the house, make food choices, and cope with discomfort, pain, and embarrassment. Lisa, my best friend and soul sister—thank you for walking through it with me. From hugs and chocolate to charcoal panty liners to filter smelly gas, you helped me find humor when I needed it most. After more than 46 years of friendship, you are still the peanut butter to my jelly—on gluten-free bread, of course.

My journey to health would not have been possible without Dr. David Hass, whose kindness and insight helped me find a path through chronic illness—thank you for being both a brilliant diagnostician and an incredible mensch. I will always be grateful.

Some of the most important turning points in my professional life began at a symposium in Boston, where I met Kate Scarlata. Through you, I also connected with the brilliant Patsy Catsos and Dr. Bill Chey and became a part of the GI nutrition community you continue to build. Your clinical wisdom and staunch and unwavering support of fellow dietitians is expansive and unmeasurable. Most of all, your friendship has meant the world to me.

When I set out to increase access to IBS nutrition, I found the incredible Julie Duffy Dillon. We met on a course about creating online courses (yes, meta!), and what began as an accountability partnership quickly turned into one of the most meaningful professional friendships of my life. Thank you for championing me, encouraging me, and bragging about me to your editor; you helped open the door to this dream.

To my editor, Rachel X. Landes—thank you for your thoughtful edits, gentle nudges, and full-throated support of my weight-inclusive approach to GI care. I am proud to be working with you and to be published by Sheldon Press.

In Chapter 7, I talk about stress management and creating your toolbox. Every Thursday at 11 am, I meet with a bunch of funny, funky, and supportive women to knit, complain, laugh, cry, and drink Starbucks. These ladies have been with me through every chapter and iteration of this book and I couldn't have written it without their support.

And finally, to my clients—thank you. You are the reason I do this work. Your resilience, your struggles, and your small victories have taught me more than any textbook ever could. Every time your symptoms improve or your quality of life gets better, I celebrate with you. And every time you continue to suffer, I dig deeper, determined to find new ways to help. You have made me a better practitioner, a better advocate, and a better human. I am forever grateful.

References

Arif, T. B. MBBS, MD1*, Ali, S. H. MBBS2, Sadiq, M. MBBS2, Bhojwani, K. D. MBBS3, Hasan, F. MD4, Rahman, A. U. MD5, and Khan, M. Z. MD6, S753, "Meta-Analysis of Global Prevalence and Gender Distribution of Irritable Bowel Syndrome (IBS) Using Rome III and IV Criteria," *The American Journal of Gastroenterology*, 119(10S): S517, October 2024. doi:10.14309/01.ajg.0001032380.70787.14

Black, C. J., Thakur, E. R., Houghton, L. A., Quigley, E. M. M., Moayyedi, P., and Ford, A. C., "Efficacy of Psychological Therapies for Irritable Bowel Syndrome: Systematic Review and Network Meta-analysis," *Gut*, 2020, 69(8): 1441–1451. doi:10.1136/gutjnl-2020-321191

Chey, W. D., Hashash, J. G., Manning, L., and Chang, L., "AGA Clinical Practice Update on the Role of Diet in Irritable Bowel Syndrome: Expert Review," *Gastroenterology*, 2022, 162(6): 1737–1745.e5. doi:10.1053/j.gastro.2021.12.248

Cong, X., Li, Y., and Bian, R., "Relationship between Neuroticism and Gastrointestinal Symptoms in Irritable Bowel Syndrome: The Mediating Role of Sleep," *Iran J Public Health*, 2022, 51(9): 1999–2006. doi:10.18502/ijph.v51i9.10554

Di Vincenzo, F., Del Gaudio, A., Petito, V., Lopetuso, L. R., and Scaldaferri, F., "Gut Microbiota, Intestinal Permeability, and Systemic Inflammation: A Narrative Review," *Intern Emerg Med*, 2024, 19(2): 275–293. doi:10.1007/s11739-023-03374-w

Halmos, E. P., and Gibson, P. R., "Controversies and Reality of the FODMAP Diet for Patients with Irritable Bowel Syndrome," *J Gastroenterol Hepatol*, 2019, 34(7): 1134–1142. doi:10.1111/jgh.14650

Janssen, P., "Can Eating Disorders Cause Functional Gastrointestinal Disorders?," *Neurogastroenterol Motil*, 2010 Dec, 22(12): 1267–1269. doi:10.1111/j.1365-2982.2010.01621.x. PMID: 21105315

Nanayakkara, W. S., Skidmore, P. M., O'Brien, L., Wilkinson, T. J., and Gearry, R. B., "Efficacy of the Low FODMAP Diet for Treating Irritable Bowel Syndrome: The Evidence to Date," *Clin Exp Gastroenterol*, 2016, 9: 131–142. doi:10.2147/CEG.S86798

Ochoa, K. C., Samant, S., Liu, A., et al., "In Vitro Efficacy of Targeted Fermentable Oligosaccharides, Disaccharides, Monosaccharides, and Polyols Enzymatic Digestion in a High-Fidelity Simulated Gastrointestinal Environment," *Gastro Hep Adv*, 2022, 2(3): 283–290. doi:10.1016/j.gastha.2022.10.011

Peters, S. L., Gibson, P. R., and Halmos, E. P., "Smartphone App-Delivered Gut-Directed Hypnotherapy Improves Symptoms of Self-Reported Irritable Bowel Syndrome: A Retrospective Evaluation," *Neurogastroenterol Motil*, 2023, 35(4): e14533. doi:10.1111/nmo.14533

Takakura, W., and Pimentel, M., "Small Intestinal Bacterial Overgrowth and Irritable Bowel Syndrome – An Update," *Front Psychiatry*, 2020, 11: 664. doi:10.3389/fpsyt.2020.00664

Trindade, I. A., Melchior, C., Törnblom, H., and Simrén, M., "Quality of Life in Irritable Bowel Syndrome: Exploring Mediating Factors Through Structural Equation Modelling," *J Psychosom Res*, 2022, 159: 110809. doi:10.1016/j.jpsychores.2022.110809

Tylka, T. L., Annunziato, R. A., Burgard, D., et al., "The Weight-Inclusive Versus Weight-Normative Approach to Health: Evaluating the Evidence for Prioritizing Well-Being over Weight Loss," *J Obes.*, 2014, 2014: 983495. doi:10.1155/2014/983495

Index